THE
GOSPEL
ALIVE

*Caring for Persons
with AIDS
and Related Illnesses*

A Pastoral Document Prepared by
The Catholic Health Association of the United States
and
The Conference of Major Religious Superiors of Men's Institutes
of the United States, Inc.

Library of Congress Cataloging-in-Publication Data

The Gospel alive: caring for persons with AIDS and related illnesses.
  p.   cm.
  Bibliography: p.
  ISBN 0-87125-149-3
  1. AIDS (Disease) — Patients — Pastoral counseling of. 2. AIDS (Disease) — Religious aspects — Catholic Church. 3. Church work with gays. 4. Pastoral medicine — Catholic Church. 5. Catholic Church — Membership. — I. Catholic Health Association of the United States. II. Conference of Major Religious Superiors of Men's Institutes of the United States.
BX2347.8.A52G67   1988
261.8'321969792 — dc19   88-14117
                                                                  CIP

Contents

Foreword

*T*oday you are faced with new challenges, new needs. One of these is the present crisis of immense proportions, which is that of AIDS and AIDS-related complex (ARC). Besides your professional contribution and your human sensitivities toward all affected by this disease, you are called to show the love and compassion of Christ and his Church. As you courageously affirm and implement your moral obligation and social responsibility to help those who suffer, *you are, individually and collectively, living out the parable of the Good Samaritan* (Lk 10:30-32).

> —Pope John Paul II
> Speech to The Catholic Health
>   Association of the United States
> Phoenix, AZ
> Sept. 14, 1987

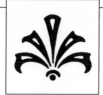

Co-Authors

Diana Bader, OP, PhD
Senior Associate
Theology, Mission and Ethics
The Catholic Health Association
 of the United States
St. Louis, MO

Roland J. Faley, TOR
Executive Director
Conference of Major Religious
 Superiors of Men's Institutes
 of the United States, Inc.
Silver Spring, MD

Mark A. Kadzielski, JD
Wiessburg & Aronson, Inc.
Los Angeles, CA

F. Daniel Krapf
Associate Vice President
Member Services
The Catholic Health Association
 of the United States
St. Louis, MO

Elizabeth McMillan, RSM, PhD
Senior Associate
Theology, Mission and Ethics
The Catholic Health Association
 of the United States
St. Louis, MO

Laurence J. O'Connell, PhD,
 STD
Vice President
Theology, Mission and Ethics
The Catholic Health Association
 of the United States
St. Louis, MO

J. Stuart Showalter, JD
Vice President
Member Services
The Catholic Health Association
 of the United States
St. Louis, MO

Introduction

"The joys and hopes, the grief and the anxiety of the
people of this age, and especially those who are poor or
in any way affected, these too are the joys and hopes,
the grief and the anxiety of the followers of Christ."
                                    Second Vatican Council

The Roman Catholic Church addresses human hopes and shares in the human condition. Thus acquired immune deficiency syndrome (AIDS), a serious problem that we have scarcely begun to address, is a matter of great concern for the Church and its ministries.

AIDS is many things. It is tragic, threatening, and cruel. For the Church, AIDS is also *kairos*—a special moment of grace and opportunity, a decisive or crucial point in time.

This book addresses AIDS in relation to the special opportunity it provides all of us, as Church, to herald Christ's message and care for others.

AIDS is tragic. There is no cure for AIDS. It inflicts overwhelming pain, complete physical disability, and severe psychological suffering on its victims. And although some treatments may temporarily arrest an illness associated with the syndrome, 70 percent of persons· with AIDS (PWAs)* die within two years of diagnosis and 100 percent die from it eventually. Strictly speaking, AIDS is not the immediate cause of death; rather, its debilitating effects on the immune system open the way for

---

*A word about usage. Many persons are, quite correctly, concerned about the appearance of depersonalization when people are referred to with acronyms. The authors are aware of and sensitive to this concern; nevertheless, "PWA" and "PWARC" are used in this text because of their convenience, because alternatives are considered demeaning (e.g.,

opportunistic diseases and infections, which are the direct causes of death.

AIDS is threatening. It threatens every segment of society. AIDS has no respect for political boundaries, race, religious beliefs, gender, or sexual orientation. All human beings—regardless of age, social status, financial means, profession, or intellectual abilities—will be affected by this devastating illness in some way. It is as menacing as the plague of 1348 or the influenza pandemic of 1918.

AIDS is cruel. Not only is AIDS fatal, but society has already stigmatized the majority of those stricken: the homosexual, the intravenous (IV) drug abuser, the prostitute. It also attacks children born of IV drug abusers or human immunodeficiency virus (HIV) carriers; men and women whose sexual partners are carriers; and people who have received infected blood products in medical treatment. (Since the discovery of the HIV test in 1985, however, the threat of acquiring AIDS through medical treatment is almost zero.)[1]

AIDS points to kairos. As the spread of AIDS takes on epidemic proportions, the Church is called to an even greater response. Every community within and outside of the Church may be touched by AIDS. Every Church ministry may be caring for PWAs at some time and assisting their families and friends to cope with this tragic illness. Every part of the Church should be helping society understand and address the complex issues surrounding AIDS.

In the face of the intense, widespread suffering that AIDS has caused, the Church's call is no less compelling than in past centuries. This is a new opportunity to live out the parable of the Good Samaritan, and since AIDS is not a sectarian issue, neither should the Church's response be sectarian. Christians and persons of other faiths have suffered from AIDS, as have those with no religious affiliation. The question that ends the parable of the Good Samaritan, "Who is my neighbor?" has only one answer: anyone in need.

"victim") or potentially inaccurate ("patient"), and because they are terms that are well accepted by both those affected with the conditions and those who care or advocate for them. In using these shorthand expressions, the authors intend no disrespect to the personhood of any individual and ask that readers understand the terms in their full meanings: "person(s) with AIDS" and "person(s) with ARC."

The Church is particularly affected because of its extensive role in the healthcare ministry. The Catholic healthcare ministry has focused primarily on care of the poor, the marginated, and the disenfranchised. This ministry has always been the leader in fulfilling unmet and poorly met needs.[2] Catholic healthcare also has always been an integral part of communities in addressing serious issues. Because of its mission and philosophy, the Catholic healthcare ministry may find that its resources are taxed to the utmost if AIDS reaches the proportions that are predicted. The complexities of AIDS, however, should awaken the Church and its ministries to the opportunities and challenges toward the PWA as well as toward society as a whole.

Whether clergy, vowed religious, or laity; whether in education, social services, or healthcare; whether a facility, system, or religious institute, our challenge is to respond to PWAs in a generous and courageous way. In so doing, we allow the healing presence of Jesus to be revealed. As persons created in the image of God, we must deal with AIDS not by reviling, judging, discriminating, and condemning, but by acting with compassion, love, justice, and mercy.

Thus the tragic, threatening, cruel condition known as AIDS is truly *kairos*—a crucial point in time and an opportunity for the Gospel of Jesus to come alive. This time also provides us with an opportunity to live out the values we espouse, to care for persons without judging by recognizing and responding to human needs as Christ would, and to acknowledge our solidarity with one another. (See Chapter 2 for a further discussion of *kairos*.)

The Catholic Health Association of the United States and the Conference of Major Religious Superiors of Men's Institutes of the United States, Inc. have prepared this book in order that those who love, work with, or care for persons with AIDS may better understand the physical illness, the complex issues associated with it, and the needs of those who have it. AIDS is a world-wide problem; however, this document addresses the United States perspective. It does not address all the issues, answer all the questions, or propose all the solutions to AIDS-related problems. Neither is it intended to question the Church's teaching on human sexuality or any other subject. Its purpose is to better inform readers about the syndrome so they will know the issues and questions and will begin to see how to devise solutions that will work in particular settings. This book also includes revised portions of two other CHA publications: *AIDS: Legal Implications for Health Care Providers* by Mark A. Kadzielski, JD, and *AIDS: Ethical Guidelines for Health Care Providers* by Diana Bader, OP, PhD, and Elizabeth McMillan, RSM, PhD.

The Gospel Alive was authorized for publication by the governing bodies of both The Catholic Health Association and the Conference of Major Religious Superiors of Men's Institutes at their respective meetings in April 1988.

We are being called to respond to the tragedy of AIDS; called to respond as Christ would; called to make the Gospel of Jesus come alive. With this book we hope to create an awareness that this devastating illness provides all of us, as Church, with a special opportunity to herald Christ's message and to care for others.

NOTES

1. *The AIDS Book. Information for Workers*, Service Employees International Union. Washington, DC, March 1986, p. 4.
2. John Michael Cox, "Justice, Compassion Needed in Treating AIDS Patients," *Health Progress*, May 1986.

1

The Facts Today

*"This sickness is not to end in death; rather it
is for God's glory, that through it the Son of God
may be glorified."*

Jn 11:4

In 1981, five young homosexual men in Los Angeles succumbed to a rare form of pneumonia from the organism *Pneumocystis carinii.* At the same time eight homosexual men in New York City were diagnosed with a rare form of cancer called Kaposi's sarcoma. As a result of reporting these cases to the Centers for Disease Control (CDC) in Atlanta, researchers soon determined that these patients had a suppression of a white blood cell that is essential to fighting infections and diseases. The CDC eventually called this new disorder *acquired immune deficiency syndrome* or AIDS.[1]

WHAT IS AIDS?

AIDS is caused by a virus recently renamed the *human immunodeficiency virus* (HIV). This was previously called human T-lymphotropic virus, type III (HTLV-III). The HIV virus infects the white blood T cells, weakening the body and destroying its natural ability to resist life-threatening diseases. Thus, destruction of the T cells breaks down the immune system, leaving the body defenseless against opportunistic infections and disease.[2]

Most of those who are HIV positive remain healthy for a time. Some only experience an elevation in temperature at the time of initial infection and remain asymptomatic.[3] Others, for reasons as yet unclear, go on to develop AIDS. The time from being infected by the HIV virus to the onset of symptoms usually ranges from six months to five years or more.

The symptoms may include:[4]

- Fever and night sweats
- Unexplained weight loss
- Diarrhea, usually severe and chronic
- Swollen lymph glands in neck, armpit, or groin areas
- White spots or blemishes in the mouth
- Fatigue
- Other manifestations may include aching joints and rashes

Ultimately, AIDS is defined as the occurrence of opportunistic diseases indicative of cell-mediated immunodeficiency in the absence of a known cause, with evidence of HIV infection.[5] Laboratory tests that demonstrate profound immune dysfunction and loss of T-4 lymphocytes support the clinical diagnosis.

Some people that are HIV positive have many of the symptoms listed but do not develop the defined characteristics of AIDS. Their condition is usually referred to as *AIDS-related complex (ARC)*. ARC can, but does not necessarily, lead to AIDS.

TESTING FOR AIDS

Testing is available to determine whether a person is carrying HIV antibodies. A positive test does not mean that the person has AIDS. Rather, this indicates that the person has been exposed to the virus. No accurate projections are available to predict the percentage of HIV-positive persons who may develop AIDS. Initial estimates put this figure at 10 percent; now an estimated 25 percent to 50 percent of HIV-positive persons may contract AIDS within 5-10 years of infection.[6] Some believe that eventually 100 percent may develop AIDS.

A negative test does not necessarily mean that a person is free of the AIDS virus. Rather, this indicates that at the time of testing, the results did not register positive. Authorities recommend that those who test negative should be retested in three to six months to confirm the negative result.

MODES OF TRANSMISSION

HIV is primarily spread through sexual contact, sharing of intravenous (IV) needles, invasive exposure to infected blood, and perinatal exposure. The virus has been found in blood, semen, vaginal secretions, saliva, tears, feces, and urine. The first three, however, are believed to be the primary sources of transmission.[7] (Recent news reports indicate some suspicion that other body fluids may also transmit the virus; this has not been confirmed, however, at the time of publication.)

Sexual transmission of the virus can occur by direct genital or rectal mucosa contact with infected semen or vaginal secretions. The virus can be transmitted through vaginal, anal, or oral intercourse. Infected males can transmit the virus to a male or female partner, and infected females can transmit the virus sexually to males and perinatally to their unborn infants.[8] HIV can also be transmitted through breast milk. Since the development in 1985 of HIV antibody testing, those receiving blood transfusions or blood products are at extremely low risk. The virus can be transmitted, however, through invasive procedures that expose persons to infected blood and, as mentioned, through sharing of IV needles.

AIDS cannot be contracted through casual contact, that is, contact that is not sexual or does not involve blood. In other words, AIDS cannot be contracted from daily contact at work, school, or home. In virtually all cases to date, AIDS has resulted from direct intimate sexual contact or sharing of needles; a few cases have been reported of medical personnel contracting AIDS through invasive contact with contaminated needles or through infected blood coming into contact with open sores or lesions; a small percentage of persons acquired it through contaminated blood or blood products in medical treatment of other illnesses.

DEMOGRAPHICS

As of December 1987, the CDC reported a cumulative total of 49,743 persons diagnosed with AIDS, with 7 percent women and 2 percent children. More than half (52 percent) of those diagnosed have died.[9] It is estimated that between 500,000 and 1.7 million persons carry the HIV infection.[10] Since no cure exists at present, all others with active cases are expected to die as a result of the condition.

When first reports were issued, 95 percent of AIDS patients were homosexual or bisexual males. Today, approximately 73 percent have acquired AIDS through homosexual or bisexual contact; IV drug users account for approximately 17 percent of cases; approximately 4 percent have contracted it through heterosexual contact; 5 percent received it through contaminated blood or blood products; and approximately 2 percent are children who acquired AIDS through infected mothers or medical treatment for another illness.[11]

The percentage of transmission from homosexual contact is expected to decline in the future as infections among children are expected to increase tenfold by 1991. New cases among heterosexuals are expected to increase to 7,000 in the same period.[12]

AIDS AMONG MINORITIES

AIDS is developing among blacks and Hispanics in numbers disproportionate to their shares of the population. As of February 1987, 25 percent of all AIDS patients were blacks (who account for 11 percent of the population) and 14 percent were Hispanics (who account for 8 percent of the population). Overall, 72 percent of all adult heterosexual men and women with AIDS are black or Hispanic. Additionally, 54 percent of all pediatric cases involve black children and 25 percent involve Hispanics. AIDS occurs 3 times more frequently among black and Hispanic men than among white men, 14 times as frequently among black women, and 9 times as frequently among Hispanic women.[13]

Black heterosexuals are actually at greater relative risk for exposure to the AIDS virus than white heterosexuals for two reasons. First, 34 percent (as of August 1987) of blacks with AIDS are IV drug abusers who pass the virus through heterosexual activity. Second, black male homosexuals may be more likely than white male homosexuals to engage in bisexual activity, often because of the strong stigma attached to homosexuality by the black community.[14]

Although AIDS among blacks has been heavily portrayed as an IV drug use problem, 39 percent of the cases (August 1987) were attributed to homosexual or bisexual transmission, 34 percent to IV drug use, and 6.7 percent to both factors. For the Hispanic population, comparable figures were 48 percent attributed to homosexual or bisexual behavior, 35 percent to IV drug abuse, and 6.6 percent to both factors.[15]

AIDS AMONG WOMEN AND CHILDREN

As of February 1988, 3,791 women and 789 children had AIDS.[16]

Most women with AIDS (78 percent) fall into two primary risk factors: IV drug users (51 percent) and heterosexual contact with an infected partner. If a woman is HIV positive or actually has the disease herself, the risk of infecting the newborn is 50 to 65 percent.[17]

Approximately 18 percent of children with AIDS acquired the infection through blood or blood products. Many were hemophiliacs, and some had open heart surgery or had transfusions as newborns.[18] Most children with the disease acquired it from their mother. Authorities suspect that some children acquired AIDS through abuse, but no data are available to indicate this at present.

The doubling time for new cases is slowing from 6 months in 1985 to 14 months in 1987.[19] The time from diagnosis to death remains at 2 years. Because of new medical treatment persons with AIDS (PWAs) are beginning to live longer.

COST OF CARE

Estimates of the cost of treating AIDS vary widely because of such factors as geography, what costs are included, and the lack of a standard treatment model. In addition, the inadequacy of outpatient and support services and the lack of reimbursement for those services can drive up the total costs of treating PWAs because of a corresponding increase in the number of inpatient days required.

The cost of care for PWAs over the duration of the syndrome is estimated at $200,000 by the medical director of the American Insurance Consultants to $67,500 by the Institute for Health Studies.[20] Current studies estimate the average annual cost at $36,000. The Public Health Service has estimated that the cost of caring for PWA's and related illnesses may rise to $16 billion by 1991.[21] Average lifetime hospital costs are now between $60,000 and $75,000; this is a result of shorter length of stay and a decrease in the number of times the AIDS patient is hospitalized. New treatments and alternative levels of care being developed are the primary reasons for this decrease.

Studies have shown that costs vary significantly according to the population served. San Francisco, with 85 percent of the white homosexual male PWA population who are not IV drug users and with a strong community-based service delivery network, has reduced average hospital inpatient stay to 12 days. The average cost for each AIDS patient in San Francisco is $27,500. New York City, on the other hand, has 45 percent of the minority PWA population in the United States, and IV drug users account for 30 percent of the city's PWAs. High medical treatment costs and absence of fully developed community-based services in New York City has kept inpatient stays at an average of 25 days and hospital costs per AIDS patient at approximately $46,500.[22]

NOTES

1. Editors, "AIDS: Responding to the Crisis," *Health Progress*, May 1986, p. 29.
2. The definition of what AIDS is was developed through multiple information sources such as: *The Latest Facts About AIDS*, American Red Cross and U.S. Public Health Service, October 1986; Ken Mayer and Hank Pizer. *The Family Guide to AIDS*, a series of Handbooks for people with AIDS, San Francisco AIDS Foundation, Revised 1987, Banton Books, 1983; C. Everett Koop, *Surgeon Generals Report on Acquired Immune Deficiency Syndrome*, U.S. Department of Health and Human Services, Washington, DC.
3. Kenneth H. Mayer, "The Clinical Challenges of AIDS and HIV Infection," *Law, Medicine and Healthcare*, Vol. 14, No. 5-6, December 1986, p. 286.
4. Symptoms were developed from multiple sources. See Note 2.
5. Nancy Mueller, "The Epidemiology of the Human Immunodeficiency Virus Infection," *Law, Medicine and Healthcare*, Vol. 14, No. 5-6, December 1986, p. 250.
6. *Confronting AIDS: Directions for Public Health, Health Care, and Research*, Institute of Medicine, National Academy of Science, National Academy Press, Washington, DC, 1986.
7. Mueller, p. 256.
8. Mueller, p. 256.
9. *Morbidity and Mortality Weekly Report*, Centers for Disease Control, Atlanta, GA, Dec. 7, 1987.
10. Michael J. Barry, Paul D. Cleary, and Harvey V. Fineberg, "Screening for HIV Infection: Risks, Benefits, and the Burden of Proof," *Law, Medicine and Healthcare*, Vol. 14, No. 5-6, December 1986, p. 259.
11. *Coping with AIDS*, Psychological and Social Considerations in Helping People with HIV-III Infection, U.S. Department of Health and Human Services, National Institute of Mental Health, Rockville, MD, 1987, p. 4.
12. *Confronting AIDS: Directions for Public Health, Health Care, and Research*, Institute of Medicine, National Academy of Science, National Academy Press, Washington, DC, 1986.

13. "Issue 1: Factors influencing AIDS Service Delivery," *AIDS Into The Nineties, Conference Working Paper,* presented at the National Network on AIDS, Washington, DC, October 1987.
14. Issue 1, *AIDS Into The Nineties.*
15. Issue 1, *AIDS Into The Nineties.*
16. *Morbidity and Mortality Weekly Report,* Centers for Disease Control, Atlanta, GA, Feb. 1, 1987.
17. Moses Grossman, "Children with AIDS," *AIDS: Principles, Practices and Politics,* Ed. by B. Corless and Mary Pittman-Lindeman, Hemisphere Publishing Corporation, New York, 1988.
18. Grossman.
19. Issue 1, *AIDS Into The Nineties.*
20. Anthony Pascal, "The Cost of Treating AIDS under Medicaid 1986-1991," The Rand Corporation, Santa Monica, CA, May 1987.
21. Issue 1, *AIDS Into The Nineties.*
22. Issue 1, *AIDS Into The Nineties.*

2

Theological Considerations

*"For I know well the plans I have for you, says the
Lord, plans for your welfare, not woe; plans to give
you a future full of hope."*

Jr 29:11

SEIZING A SACRED MOMENT

We believe God has a plan for the salvation of all people. That plan
began to unfold explicitly among the Hebrews, reached its full potential
in Jesus Christ, and now strives for completion in the Christian Church.
This is the history of salvation. It behooves the Christian community to
remember this understanding of history in times of crisis—e.g. the AIDS
crisis.

We also believe God acts in history, offering us signs of saving
presence. As believers, we await these signs, these special moments of
visitation, with confident assurance. They often emerge as events within
the ebb and flow of everyday experience, and there is always a double
message. On their face they may seem either threatening or inviting. We
are reassured of the loving God's saving presence and are reminded that
the community of believers, the Church, must exemplify to the world the
qualities of the loving God—qualities of goodness, generosity, fidelity,
forgiveness, beauty, and mercy.

We believe as well that "at all times the Church carries the
responsibility of reading the signs of the time and of interpreting them in
the light of the Gospel, if it is to carry on its task."[1] Thus, the Church is
responsible for surveying the sweep of human experience; it must "discern
in the events, the needs, and the longings which it shares with other men

and women of our time, what may be genuine signs of the presence or of the purpose of God."[2] In short, the Church has been commissioned to discern and draw attention to those special moments in history when God's presence and concern are especially evident.

KAIROS

Significant moments in the Judeo-Christian tradition have been referred to as *kairos*, that is, a decisive or crucial place or point in time. *Kairos* precipitates a turning point. It is a time when God makes available the possibility of radical transformation. *Kairos*, then, connotes a specific situation that demands a decision on the part of individuals or the community. *Kairos* refers to those special moments when God draws near, demanding recognition and response. When salvation history makes itself forcefully felt in the theater of ordinary human experience, we have *kairos*.

The incarnation of Jesus Christ is the ultimate example of *kairos*. In Jesus, God dramatically broke into human experience, identified with it, and placed demands on it. Indeed, the Christ-event was a time of special visitation. It was *kairos par excellence*, and with it the reign of God drew near (Mk 1:15). Jerusalem, however, did not recognize this unique *kairos* when Jesus announced it (Lk 19:44), and thus we see that *kairos* is not always self-evident. The decisive character of an event or moment (*kairos*) must be discerned.

This underscores the importance of the Church in clearly identifying the "signs of the time," that is, in recognizing and drawing attention to the *kairos*-character of specific moments in the history of the human family. In identifying a given situation as a particularly expectant moment for the recognition of God among us, the Church also assumes a responsibility for acting creatively to make visible this invisible presence.

Jesus emphasized the action-oriented nature of *kairos* when, at the beginning of his passion, he said: "My time is near" (Mt. 26:18). Throughout his life the *kairos*-character of Jesus' mission emerged with increasing clarity. His suffering, death, and resurrection constituted the ultimate, visible witness to the love of God in human history. Thus Christians, like Christ, are called to recognize *kairos* and to fulfill concretely its demands through acts that allow the presence of God to shine forth. *Kairos* is a call to action.

THE AIDS CRISIS: CURSE OR KAIROS?

The AIDS virus is indeed a curse. When it takes hold of the human body, it must be presumed to be fatal in all cases. However, persons suffering from AIDS are neither cursed nor are they a curse, they are—simply—ill.

Certainly nothing inherently good exists in the scourge of AIDS, but it does draw attention to our own responsibility. It is a powerful sign of the times that should elicit a positive response. It would not be stretching a point, therefore, to characterize this moment in history as *kairos*-charged. It is a reminder to the Christian community that we must exemplify the qualities of the loving God by recognizing in the AIDS crisis an extraordinary opportunity, a special time to care and act.

Pope John Paul II was unequivocal in characterizing AIDS as a special situation that challenges the Church to be true to its identity as a sign of God's love and concern:

> Besides your professional contribution and your human sensitivities toward all affected by this disease, you are called to show the love and compassion of Christ and his Church . . . to express love, solidarity and service, and to exclude selfishness, discrimination, and neglect.[3]

Thus the AIDS crisis is a profound challenge to the Church. It will force us to live out our Christian identity with renewed vigor, and it will drive us to a deeper understanding of the practical demands of that identity in our own times. The AIDS epidemic will shake many foundations, but this should not be surprising. *Kairos* was not meant to be comfortable, but rather to be the new point in time when God works creatively. As the instruments of that creativity, we must act courageously and with quiet confidence, always remembering the words of Jesus: "I will be with you until the end of time" (Mk 28:20).

NOTES

1. Vatican II, *Gaudium et Spes*, 905.
2. *Gaudium et Spes*.
3. Pope John Paul II, "Address to the Catholic Health Care Ministry," *Health Progress*, November 1987, p. 15.

3

The Church and Society

"I give you a new commandment:
Love one another:
Such as my love has been for you
so must your love be for each other.
This is how all will know you for my disciples:
by your love for one another."

Jn 13:34-35

Whether we are members of the Church, or are part of a human social service organization, or are acting on our own in responding to AIDS, we are part of the larger complex group that is our society.

By definition, members of a society do not function independently of one another; a society is made up of interdependent groups: political, governmental, neighborhood, church, school, familial, etc. Each of these groups forms "community," groupings of people with a sense of "belonging" and with similar customs, values, and ideals. Each subset of community has its way of looking at life and addressing issues, problems, and concerns. The ways various communities bond together greatly influence the outcome of contemporary issues, and because all elements of society are affected by AIDS, our collective reaction to AIDS and to persons with AIDS (PWAs) is influenced by the attitudes of each segment of society.[1]

SPECIAL ISSUES AND NEEDS

In addressing the plethora of complex AIDS issues that face us as a society, we are seemingly overwhelmed by the strong moral and psychological components that the illness presents. AIDS has an obvious relationship to behaviors that are not present in most other illnesses.[2] Among PWAs, the vast majority are male homosexuals or IV drug abusers; the majority of afflicted women are IV drug abusers or prostitutes. Because persons already stigmatized are those most affected, moralizing and discriminatory attitudes create new suffering that goes beyond the physical effects.

Growing numbers of heterosexuals are also contacting AIDS, particularly women whose sexual partners knowingly or unknowingly are in the high-risk group. Infected women are also bearing children with AIDS. Theoretically, every member of our society is at risk for contracting the illness if they engage in high-risk behaviors or engage in sex with those who are in the high-risk categories.[3] Our communities and society may lose the talents of many leaders, mothers and fathers, educators, artists, and others, before the AIDS crisis is over.

A deeply pastoral and compassionate response is needed to address the issues surrounding AIDS. Every subgroup in society must work together to overcome negative attitudes, fear, and biases about AIDS and PWAs.[4] The Church and its ministries, especially Catholic healthcare, can be vital in understanding and responding to such factors as:

- The needs of homosexuals to be active participants in the community
- The plight of the IV drug abusers and what may cause persons to seek drugs
- The needs of impoverished women who turn to drugs or prostitution
- The pain connected with disclosure of sexual orientation or life style
- The devastating feeling of rejection or alienation from God, Church, family, and friends
- The real and unreal fears of people in relation to the illness and its transmission
- The moral dimension of the medical advice regarding prevention (use of condoms, "safe sex," etc.)
- The physical and psychological pain caused by AIDS and the various modes of treatment
- The conflict between the rights of the individual and those of society with regard to mandatory testing, quarantining, etc.
- Issues of confidentiality and privacy

- Issues of funding for care of PWAs
- Questions regarding pastoral responsibilities toward the PWA, the family, associates, and those who live in fear of the illness
- Issues on quality of care
- The uneven distribution of programs and services to meet the needs of PWAs and others
- The struggle to overcome the mentality that AIDS is "God's punishment"

All of these are issues for society, as well as for the Catholic Church and its ministries, which can be initiators and influencers in resolving them. Admittedly, they may not be easily resolved; however, by addressing and resolving these issues, we may be creating the template for resolving even larger issues of society.

Many factors in the AIDS crisis require moral guidance that goes beyond the Church's often-stated norms on sexual ethics. Such guidance should deal with the reflexive, homophobic attitudes and simplistic ideas of moral retribution that some persons hold with regard to AIDS. Traditional principles of Christian morality remain valid, but today's complex issues and questions arising from AIDS require other approaches and answers as well.

The Church, as a vital force in society, has an important agenda to join with other groups in society to call for a cure for AIDS. Until a cure is found, however, the agenda calls for addressing and resolving other conflicts generated by the AIDS crisis.

NEGATIVE ATTITUDES AND FEAR

A major social issue in the AIDS tragedy is the negative, often hostile, attitudes that surround homosexuals, IV drug abusers, and prostitutes; AIDS appears to be an opportunity to lash back.[5] These attitudes have greatly affected our response to AIDS and to PWAs: government has been slow to respond with funds for research; some persons advocate legislation to quarantine or further isolate these groups; and groups believe that AIDS is God's punishment.

Fear compounds these negative attitudes: fear concerning AIDS and its transmission; fear for the erosion of society's moral values; fear of the overwhelming implications for public policy, resource allocation, employment, etc.; and fear about the lack of a cure.[6] Some persons and their fear have banned children with AIDS from classrooms, barred families from church, beaten up homosexuals, and in one instance burned a family's home because their children had AIDS.

Regardless of their nature and basis in fact, these fears and attitudes are real concerns, and we must address them if we are to resolve the AIDS crisis. It is the responsibility of every member of society to become knowledgeable about AIDS, to put aside biases, and to address these issues in a compassionate, intelligent, and effective manner. It is the responsibility of the Church to unite as community, to work together, and to live out the Gospel. The Gospel empowers and calls us to address AIDS openly and compassionately, to heal, to teach, and to ensure that justice, love, and mercy are reflected in public policy and teaching. Heeding the call of the Gospel and embued with the power it contains, the Church has a rich tradition of responding to catastrophic illnesses and meeting the needs of the poor, the powerless, and the disenfranchised. AIDS is an opportunity to add to that tradition.

To accept the empowerment and call of the Gospel, we as Church should work with others who are empowered. This calls for collaboration with the lawmakers, healthcare providers, payors of care, political leaders, and other decision makers to ensure adequate funding for research and care, to provide the full continuum of services, and to address not only the need for a cure but solutions to the problems of society that have caused AIDS to become so rampant.[7] Although AIDS is a challenge to society as a whole, it is particularly a challenge for us as Church in society.

NOTES

1. Eileen P. Flynn, *AIDS A Catholic Call for Compassion*, Sheed and Ward, Kansas City, MO, 1985.
2. *Coping with AIDS*, Psychological and Social Considerations in Helping People with HTLV-III Infection. U.S. Department of Health and Human Services, National Institute of Mental Health, Rockville, MD, 1986.
3. Nancy Mueller, "The Epidemiology of the Human Immunodeficiency Virus Infection," *Law, Medicine and Healthcare*, Vol 14, No. 5-6, December 1986, p. 251; Flynn.
4. Flynn.
5. Clare Ansberry, "Fear and Loathing, AIDS, Stirring Panic and Prejudice, Test the Nations Character." *The Wall Street Journal*, Vol. LXIX, No. 13, 1987.

6. Flynn, p. 24; and Leon Eisenberg, "The Genesis of Fear: AIDS and the Public Response to Science, *Law, Medicine and Healthcare,* Vol 14, No. 5-6, December 1986, p. 243-247.
7. From CHA testimony on *The Many Faces of AIDS: A Gospel Response,* before the Episcopal Task Force of National Conference of Catholic Bishops, Washington, DC, July 1987.

4

Caring for Persons with AIDS or Related Illness

"Each of them is Jesus in distressing disguise."
Mother Teresa

The Scriptures are clear about Jesus' posture before those on the periphery of society, and the Church has a longstanding tradition of presence and support for these persons. As mentioned, the person with AIDS (PWA) is today's counterpart to the Scripture's disenfranchised. Like the leper in biblical times, the PWA suffers not only the debilitating physical effects, but often faces ostracism, unwarranted fear from others, and isolation, as well as possible homophobic sentiments.

What would be Jesus' response to the pain, stress, and misunderstanding surrounding PWAs? Jesus touched the neediest: the paralytic, the elderly deformed lady, the sorrowing mother at Naim, the possessed person, and the Samaritan leper. He not only served the neediest but dined with publicans and sinners, the rejects of society. His teaching paralleled his action. It was the lost son, the lost sheep, and the lost coin that gave expression to his unbounded concern for the most abandoned (Lk 15).

In that same spirit, the Church reads the signs of the time and sees in the PWA a Gospel summons. The response should be generous and unquestioning, not cautious, delayed, or halfhearted. If they are to live up to the Gospel message, Christians cannot stand idly by while other humanitarian agencies move forward. Time is of the essence. The Church should begin immediately to galvanize its medical and pastoral resources if it is to be an effective and compassionate presence in the AIDS tragedy.

HIV TESTING AND COUNSELLING

Compassionate care begins when persons seek human immunodeficiency virus (HIV) testing, either voluntarily because they believe they are at risk or at the request of a medical professional because AIDS is suspected as the cause of illness. Health professionals need to be sensitive to the fears and anxieties of the person being tested. Counselling should begin at the time of testing.

Wherever the testing takes place, the individual must be informed about the test and the test results. First, as noted earlier, a negative test result does not necessarily mean that the person is free of AIDS; retesting should be done in three to six months to confirm the negative result. Second, a positive test result does not mean that the person has AIDS or will contract it;[1] no reliable projections exist regarding the percentage of HIV-positive persons who may develop AIDS or AIDS-related complex (ARC).

Regardless of the test result, the primary focus of counselling should be the need to change established sexual or drug habits. Those who test positive should know that they are potentially infectious to others and will presumably remain so the rest of their lives. They should understand their moral responsibility to contact past and present sexual and/or drug partners.[2] They also should receive up-to-date information about AIDS, its transmission, available treatments, and sources of care and support.

Counselling should be clear and nonjudgmental. The client should be told that the only sure way to stop the spread of AIDS is through abstinence and that "safe sex" is a misnomer.

Persons who test HIV positive may suffer stress and anxiety out of fear that they will contract AIDS. They should be given names of appropriate resources that can assist them in coping. These resources may be community-based organizations specifically formed to provide mental health, nutrition, medical, and support services to such persons.[3]

Persons who test HIV positive also should be counselled to inform their physicians, dentist, and sexual partners as well as others who may be treating them. Not informing them may be placing them at risk. Those who are informed must respect the trust that has been placed in them.[4]

CONFIDENTIALITY

Persons seeking testing should be assured at all times of confidentiality. They know they are at risk for possible discrimination or retribution if others know that they are HIV positive.

Persons being treated for AIDS or ARC should have their privacy respected. Once treatment begins, however, it may be impossible to maintain absolute confidentiality because proper treatment may create a legitimate need to know.[5] Staff caring for AIDS/ARC patients should be educated regarding the need for confidentiality and privacy.

For example, a violation of confidentiality occurred when a nurse caring for a PWA went home and told her husband that his former high school classmate was gay and had AIDS. The husband in turn told other friends. Although the husband ultimately was very supportive of his friend, the PWA was initially depressed and concerned about other friends learning he was gay.

SPECIAL CARE CONCERNS

Persons with AIDS or with ARC (PWARC) have an ongoing need for intensive medical, psychological, social, and spiritual support services. For example, they often contemplate suicide because they know AIDS is, as of now, 100 percent fatal.[6] They also know:

- AIDS is painful and debilitating
- AIDS causes not only physical deterioration but severe psychological and organic brain impairment
- Its associated illnesses causes loss of muscle and psychomotor control, seizures, impaired vision, and dementia
- Its array of opportunistic infections will eventually affect their ability to work and be independent and active in their community

Compounding these physical effects are the psychological problems caused by the HIV virus invading the brain cells. These organic changes may confuse therapists because they appear to have a psychological basis. The effect on the central nervous system may lead to confusion, seizures, and dementia; the true psychological consequences of AIDS cannot be underestimated. Persons with AIDS or ARC often undergo intense feelings of guilt or depression about their behavior and the fact that they may have infected others. Anxiety may manifest itself in physical symptoms that the patient believes are signs of AIDS-related illness. Some have even noted that the PWARCs may demonstrate more psychological distress than the PWAs because of their fear that they will develop AIDS.

MORE THAN A GAY DISEASE

Some are surprised to learn that AIDS is growing rapidly among nonhomosexuals. For example, the disease is becoming more and more prevalent among women, and women with AIDS do not fit the men's profile. Physiological, psychological and sociopolitical differences emerge when caring for women.[7] They are primarily poor and black (53 percent) or Hispanic and are single parents with families to support. Once diagnosed as being HIV positive or having AIDS or ARC, they face complex fertility and reproductive ethical dilemmas.[8] Many may be pregnant or may confront the issue of becoming pregnant. Those who are pregnant have a 50 to 65 percent chance of infecting their unborn children.[9] Pregnancy also has a serious effect on the woman's already depressed immunological system, making her even more susceptible to opportunistic infections and diseases.

These women must also cope with caring for their children as well as planning for their children's care in the event of their death. For reasons yet unknown, women die sooner from AIDS than men.[10]

Women with AIDS are often alone and in need of numerous support services. Because of their physical condition, family responsibilities, and financial constraints, however, they usually are not able to obtain the services they need.

The number of children with AIDS is also rising dramatically. Children acquire the infection primarily through transmission from the mother, either during gestation or from breast milk.

Infected infants usually begin showing signs of AIDS at about eight months.[11] Many also suffer from drug addiction because they have mothers who are drug addicts themselves. Pediatric AIDS patients are significantly more expensive to treat, have infections and diseases different from those of the adult, and require considerably longer hospitalizations. Children with AIDS usually cannot be treated and cared for at home because their mothers typically are poor and have AIDS or ARC also. It is virtually impossible to place these children in foster homes, so they are literally warehoused in hospitals until they die.[12] The hospital staff members in effect become their mothers and fathers — their family.

SOCIAL AND EMOTIONAL ISSUES

Persons with AIDS or ARC also are confronted with many social, emotional, and practical concerns. For the first time many of them must deal with their family, friends, or employer learning of their previously hidden life style.[13] Many have been shunned by relatives and friends. They may face being fired, becoming disabled, and being unable to care for themselves. They often are not able to maintain their homes or apartments, and the high cost of treatment is an extreme burden.

Their financial problems may be compounded by other factors. For example, Medicare requires a two year wait for disability coverage, and Medicaid requires PWAs to spend their savings and possibly sell their homes. PWARCs experience greater frustration because their illnesses are not in the definite AIDS category, and therefore they are not eligible for disability or some support services or treatment programs.

The attitudes of some communities where PWAs live also add to the stress. They may suffer further isolation and physical or verbal abuse when others discover they have AIDS. Some PWAs have been barred from restaurants, churches, schools, and similar places. Others have been refused emergency transportation service to hospitals. Some have had their lives threatened and their property damaged or destroyed. Some have been refused medical treatment, even in life-threatening emergencies.

These negative experiences are not universal, however. Many PWAs have experienced much love and support during their illnesses because families and friends have helped them cope. Some employers have guaranteed continued employment; others have continued health insurance coverage until the PWA is eligible for disability.

PASTORAL CARE

Pastoral care is an important component in the care of the PWA and PWARC, and it should also be extended to the person who is HIV positive. Pastoral care personnel should understand how AIDS is different from other diseases that they encounter. They should remember that they are dealing with persons who feel stigmatized, isolated, and alienated.

Absolutely essential in ministering to the person with AIDS is to offer nonjudgmental care and aid. Gaining the confidence and trust of PWAs may take time, even weeks.[14] Many do not have a church affiliation because they feel alienation from God and church because of their life style.

It is important to help the PWA and PWARC to "get in touch" with their feelings about themselves, their condition, their families and friends, and their isolation.[15] After the initial shock and depression that often follow the diagnosis, many PWAs and PWARCs experience a strong sense of spirituality. During this period they may reflect positively on their own values, their relationships with others, and the contributions they have made during their lives. This may lead to opportunities to heal torn relationships and may renew their strength to fight the disease as long as possible. Pastoral care personnel have been instrumental in helping create these positive attitudes, and many of them have reported that they themselves have received strength and courage from caring for PWAs.[16]

Time with the PWA or PWARC may be nonverbal, such as simple touching or a caring presence. Winning their trust is vital to being able to share feelings. Developing a sense of integrity will lead to more openness. Rather than acting as savior, the pastoral caregiver should have an attitude of genuine empathy, compassion, and concern without proselytizing.

The pastoral caregiver will likely deal with the PWA's family, who may encounter some of the same feelings and emotions as the PWA: anger, guilt, fear, stigma, and alienation. The caregiver will also confront issues of healing and reconciliation, since many families may be discovering the PWA's life style for the first time. In all of these areas, pastoral care can be instrumental in developing self-worth, acceptance, spiritual growth, healing, and unity for the PWA, the family, and other involved persons. At the same time, however, confidentiality must be respected.

SUPPORT SERVICES

Paramount in the care of PWAs and PWARCs, and HIV-positive persons is a good support care system. Until recently, the primary form of care has been the acute care facility, but with new treatments the length of hospital stay is decreasing. Therefore, a demand now exists for new kinds of services, with emphasis on community-based networks.

Community-based organizations (CBOs) have developed not only to provide education but also to offer direct care and treatment services. Many of these CBOs have been formed by gay organizations in major metropolitan areas. They have helped PWAs and PWARCs to stay independent as long as possible, and they have truly become the good Samaritans of the AIDS epidemic. They offer such services as counselling, legal assistance, aid in applying for Medicare or Medicaid, and advocacy. In addition, they provide financial assistance for drugs, treatment, food, and housing. Some CBOs have developed hospice and intermediate housing programs and the "buddy program," which assigns a person to be companion to a PWA or PWARC.

CBO services are available to all those afflicted with AIDS, not just gay persons. But those who are not homosexual have hesitated to use them because of the "gay stigma." In addition, it has been difficult to integrate minority groups into the CBO network. Many members of these groups are difficult to reach through normal channels, and many distrust government or white-sponsored organizations. Their access to healthcare is hindered by limited community medical resources and lack of knowledge of supportive care networks.[17] Blacks and Hispanics have not used supportive care programs extensively and often have delayed seeking medical treatment until late in the stages of the disease. (This may explain why the time from diagnosis to death is much shorter among minorities than among whites.)

As the AIDS epidemic expands into a greater proportion of the population, more CBOs will be needed. These organizations may begin to compete with one another for the limited funds available, and some believe that the minorities will have even less access to them. At present, a primary demand is to develop CBOs that can relate to and meet the education, care, and treatment needs of the minority population.[18]

NOTES

1. *The AIDS Book: Information for Workers*, Service Employees International Union, Washington, DC, March 1986, p. 6.
2. *Coping with AIDS*, Psychological and Social Considerations in Helping People with HTLV-III Infection, U.S. Department of Health and Human Services, National Institute of Mental Health, Rockville, MD.
3. *Coping with AIDS*.

4. *Coping with AIDS.*
5. John Michael Cox, "Justice, Compassion Needed in Treating AIDS Patients," *Health Progress,* May 1986., p. 34.
6. *Coping with Aids.*
7. Julian S. Murphy, "Women with AIDS: Sexual Ethics in an Epidemic," *AIDS: Principles, Practices and Politics,* Ed. by Inge B. Corless and Mary Pittman-Lindeman, Hemisphere Publishing, New York, 1988, p. 66.
8. Murphy.
9. Moses Grossman, "Children with AIDS," *AIDS: Principles, Practices, and Politics,* Ed. Inge B. Corless and Mary Pittman-Lindeman. Hemisphere Publishing Corporation, New York, 1988. p. 168.
10. Murphy, p. 66.
11. Grossman, p. 168.
12. Grossman.
13. *Coping with AIDS.*
14. Mary E. Johnson, "A Case Study in Pastoral Counselling," *Health Progress,* May 1986, p. 10.
15. Rev. Leo Tibesar, "Pastoral Care: Helping Patients on an Inward Journey," *Health Progress,* May 1986, p. 43.
16. Bernard Brown, "Creative Acceptance: Am Ethics for AIDS," *AIDS: Principles, Practices, and Politics,* Ed. Inge B. Corless and Mary Pittman-Lindeman. Hemisphere Publishing Corporation, New York, 1988, pp. 221-235.
17. Issue 4: "Forming Partnerships, Linkages, and Networks," *AIDS Into The Nineties, Conference Working Paper,* presented at the National Network on AIDS, Washington, DC, October 1987.
18. Issue 4, *AIDS Into The Nineties.*

5

The Healthcare Community

"I tell you most solemnly,
whoever believes in me
will perform the same works as I do myself,
he will perform even greater work
because I am going to the Father."

Jn 14:12

The healthcare community, particularly Catholic healthcare, has always responded heroically to epidemics and catastrophic diseases. AIDS is just such an epidemic. Not only does it have potentially catastrophic proportions, but it carries enormous implications for the healthcare system as well.[1] As discussed earlier, the medical issues are compounded by the syndrome's lethal nature, by its mode of transmission, and by a wide array of political, social, ethical, and environmental issues and concerns.

Healthcare facilities and healthcare providers have always been expected to accept a certain risk of disease as an occupational hazard. As the highly contagious and universally fatal nature of AIDS became known, however, institutions and employees became extremely fearful of the risks involved in caring for PWAs and PWARCs. This fear has carried over to IV drug users and homosexuals because they may be unknown carriers of the virus. Some healthcare workers have flatly refused to care for the PWA or PWARC.[2]

It is unethical not to care for persons with AIDS, persons with ARC, and persons in high risk groups. The healthcare community's fears and concerns, therefore, must be dealt with honestly, openly, and realistically. If they are not, it will affect not only medical care but also the development of programs and services needed in the continuum of care.

Failure to address these concerns will also aggravate the existing negative attitudes and discrimination concerning the two major high-risk groups, homosexuals and IV drug users.

FINANCIAL CONSIDERATIONS

The acute care hospital has been the primary source of service to AIDS patients. To some extent, this has created a view of AIDS as being a *medical* problem rather than a *community* problem.[3] This view creates a twofold conflict: (1) financing and reimbursement programs are based on acute care services, and, (2) development of community-based services is impeded because funding is either nonexistent or minimal.[4] As a result, hospitals have borne the burden of caring for AIDS patients; length of stay may be longer because of the lack of community-based services; and the PWA may be denied the care of more appropriate settings that enhance wellness and independence.

The financial implications of hospitals treating PWAs and PWARCs cannot be overstated. The associated illnesses of the syndrome makes AIDS very complex and costly to treat. Inadequate reimbursement, both private and governmental, has caused some healthcare facilities and organizations to be slow in responding to needs. Treating AIDS patients has affected the financial viability of many organizations.

Many AIDS patients are eligible for Medicaid but Medicaid reimbursement differs from state to state, usually falls far short of covering the actual cost of care, and tends to reimburse only for acute care rather than for community-based services. Facilities that care for large numbers of PWAs therefore encounter serious financial problems. In addition to this high cost of care, serious staffing, political, and community relations problems have also caused some organizations to delay in accepting PWAs for treatment. Reimbursement is a major issue that will have to be addressed for the sake of healthcare institutions, community organizations, and the PWAs and PWARCs. Despite the financial difficulties, many healthcare facilities have responded very well in meeting the needs. In undertaking this burden, some of these facilities have emerged as regional, state, and national leaders.

Hospitals and other institutions who have made the decision to care for PWAs and PWARCs have addressed such important issues as:

- Continuing staff education about AIDS and AIDS-related concerns
- Ensuring that well-developed infection control policies are fully understood and carried out by all staff members
- Developing personnel and medical staff policies to deal with persons refusing to care for PWAs
- Developing policies to deal with employees who test HIV positive or who have AIDS or ARC
- Involving every level of management staff in treatment and education programs
- Being a resource to the community on AIDS education and service needs

As healthcare facilities become involved in caring for PWAs, the staffing, financial, management, medical staff, and community relations issues may not be easily resolved. In larger communities the burden of care has fallen on public and teaching hospitals. As a result, many public hospitals are finding that they may not be able to survive because of the burdens placed on them by large numbers of PWAs. Similarly, some teaching hospitals that care for many PWAs are discovering that many of their residency program positions are going vacant as a result of caring for large numbers of AIDS patients. Therefore, it is important for institutions to take an active role in public education and to counteract the myths about AIDS and its transmission.

These situations raise several questions. Is it just the responsibility of a few hospitals to care for AIDS patients, or is it a community responsibility? Is it better to develop "Centers of Excellence" at a few institutions rather than spread the expertise over many? If a few facilities are caring for AIDS patients and are having problems surviving, should it not become a community healthcare issue to help support these institutions as they meet the challenges this epidemic requires?

Beyond these issues, institutions have found that once PWAs are admitted, treated, and stabilized, there may be nowhere to send them. For example, in one case, a PWA remained in the hospital five months longer than needed because no family member, friend, nursing home, hospice, or other facility would take him. Because he had no place to go, he remained there until he died. The patient received excellent care from the hospital staff, but they were frustrated because they knew he did not belong in a hospital and needed different support than medical care. The discharge planning staff was unable to find any nursing home within the entire state until five days before the patient died. Because that facility was 350 miles away, however, the patient's invalid father refused to have him sent so far because he did not want his son to die alone.

This case is not atypical. As this story indicates, it is virtually impossible in many communities to place a person with AIDS. Nursing homes have received much criticism, some of which may be justified; however, most nursing homes are simply not equipped for the care and treatment of persons with AIDS especially PWAs with psychological and neurological symptoms. Caring for PWAs requires special staff, equipment, and training that most nursing homes are not able to provide.

Those facilities willing to care for PWAs face the same reimbursement shortfalls and family and patient relations issues that hospitals encounter. They also may note that the PWAs feel isolated and confined to their rooms because the facilities do not have enough programs to meet their specific needs. Thus many institutions that do care for AIDS patients often consider having a unit specifically designated to caring for PWAs.

NEED FOR COMMUNITY SERVICES

If the primary burden of caring for PWAs is to be taken off the hospital, then community-based service delivery networks must be developed. The goal of such a network should be to keep AIDS patients out of the hospital and in programs that allow for independence and dignity. This requires that hospitals, nursing homes, community-based organizations (CBOs), social service agencies, etc., develop formal partnerships, alliances, and other types of linkages that break down barriers of competition and "turfism" to address the well-being of the community and the patient.

A well-planned and developed community-based service network must involve physicians.[5] At present, in most communities only a small number of physicians are treating PWAs and PWARCs, and the physicians tend to refer patients to the hospital rather than to other service networks. Physicians should be educated about what services are available and should refer patients to these organizations.

Currently, except for acute care and clinical needs, most community resources are fragmented, loosely organized and developed, and not well coordinated. In some major metropolitan areas such as San Francisco, New York, and Minneapolis, however, some excellent models of community service networks provide home health, hospice, intermediate housing, financial assistance, support groups, and many other services to meet the needs of persons with AIDS, ARC, or positive HIV tests, as well as their families, friends, and caregivers. These networks were generally started by the gay community. Hospitals, nursing homes, and other providers should use them as resources to expand their own programs. Other communities can contact these organizations for guidance and direction as they undertake to develop comprehensive services.

As discussed earlier, a serious problem in almost all communities is that CBOs and other organizations have not addressed the needs of blacks and Hispanics. IV drug users are not organized, are difficult to reach, and do not have advocates who readily address their concerns. Partnerships and networks need to address these needs or create new services that acknowledge these groups.

KEY CHALLENGES TO ADDRESS

The healthcare community must work together in addressing many problem areas as it searches for a realistic, effective response to AIDS. Such problem areas include the following:

- The PWA's special care needs, especially for psychological and mental health services.[6]
- The special education and training needs of the healthcare facility's staff.
- The necessity of having support groups to enable staff, family, and friends to deal with the emotional, psychological, and physical demands placed on *them* in caring for AIDS patients.
- The need for continuity of services both within and among healthcare facilities and with CBOs.
- The PWA's and others' need for pastoral care to heal the spiritual wounds caused by alienation from family, friends, Church, and God.

- The need to avoid "turfism" by creating coalitions among private and public agencies.
- The consideration that as treatments improve and begin to extend lives, patients may need healthcare longer and require a variety of support services.
- The need for alternative care programs, especially for those with psychological symptoms and organic brain deterioration.

Will we find solutions for these problems? The answer is difficult, but clearly we should be prepared to care for PWAs with dignity and to provide a quality of life that enables them to function as independently as possible.[7] The AIDS crisis will present new financial, ethical, and treatment issues that we should anticipate now. We should not wait for these to surface before resolving them.

In beginning to anticipate and address these challenges, we may discover many opportunities for leaders of healthcare institutions, social service agencies, churches, and civic communities to work together. Services should be well planned and coordinated. Where reimbursement is poor or nonexistent, we should develop it; where services are weak or unavailable, we should create them. No one organization has the responsibility to do all that is needed. The AIDS challenge is the responsibility of society as a whole.

NOTES

1. C. Everett Koop, "Message from the Surgeon General," *Provider*, May 1987, p. 7.
2. "Employment Issues Dominate Hospital AIDS Suit," *Hospitals*, August 20, 1987, p. 49.
3. Issue 4: Forming Partnerships, Linkages, and Networks," *AIDS Into The Nineties, Conference Working Paper*, presented at the National Network on AIDS, Washington, DC, October 1987.
4. Issue 4, *AIDS Into The Nineties*.
5. Issue 4, *AIDS Into The Nineties*.
6. *Coping with AIDS*, Psychological and Social Considerations in Helping People with HTLV-III Infection, U.S. Department of Health and Human Services, National Institute of Mental Health, Rockville, MD, 1986.
7. *Coping with AIDS*.

6

AIDS Within the Church

"Your pain is the breaking of the shell that encloses
your understanding."

Kahil Gibran

AIDS not only affects the Church in society but also touches the Church deeply within when it infects a vowed religious, a priest, or an individual preparing for religious life or the priesthood. The status of the PWA within the Church adds to the pain and stress on the affected individual as well as on the person's religious superior or bishop and the religious or Church community.

The AIDS-related issues and concerns that face major superiors and bishops are numerous, have no simple answers, and will affect major policy decisions of the religious order or diocese. This section addresses some of the key issues, concerns, and questions that may surface in making such policies.

EDUCATION PROGRAM

All members of a religious or diocesan community should be educated and prepared for the eventuality that one of their own may develop AIDS. A priority in major policy decisions is that religious and clergy should know and understand what AIDS is, how it is contracted, and how it affects the individual physically, psychologically, and emotionally. Beyond the effects on the PWA, they also must deal with how the situation may influence their relationship with the PWA personally and within the community.

An educational program should include the importance of dealing with emotions, that range from total support to anger, betrayal, or embarrassment and dealing with people who are judgmental and condemning. Although these feelings and responses are understandable, particularly if AIDS was contracted not as a result of treatment for illness but through sexual activity, they are, nevertheless, factors that must be confronted. Major superiors and bishops have the responsibility to reinforce their members in a chaste and celebate life in keeping with their commitment.

The AIDS education program for clergy and religious also should address sexuality openly and frankly. Our sexual nature is one of God's gifts, and it is not easily denied or suppressed. Sexuality of religious and clergy carries with it the same issues of vulnerability and humanness as it does for anyone else. The education program should strive to create a greater understanding of our sexual nature and how one can best deal with it within religious or clerical life.

TESTING FOR AIDS

- Should HIV testing be required of all persons requesting admission into a religious institute or the seminary?
- What are the motivating factors requiring a policy of mandatory testing?
- Is testing required to better help applicants understand the implications for themselves of being HIV positive and the possible effects on their ability to serve the Church in ministry?

Regardless of whether HIV testing is required, applicants must understand the demands and stresses of dedicating themselves to life within the Church. Great physical, emotional, and spiritual stamina is required. Any serious illness could affect one's ability to cope with the multidimensional rigors of the religious vocation. Being HIV positive may not itself affect an individual's ability to fulfill the responsibilities to ministry; however, the stress of knowing that one is HIV positive could impede the person's ability to cope with the everyday stresses of carrying out one's ministry.

Is testing desired to avoid high costs of future care? If this is the case, it should be noted that very soon technology will be available to predict an individual's predisposition to certain cancers, heart disease, and other devastating and costly illnesses. Although the cost of care is an important consideration, it should not be the sole determining factor in establishing an AIDS testing policy.

As already emphasized in other sections, testing for the HIV antibodies is not entirely reliable and is not determinative of whether the person will or will not develop AIDS or ARC. A negative result only means that, at the time of testing, the individual has not produced antibodies that would indicate a positive result. A positive result may also be inconclusive since a small but significant percentage of false positives have been reported for this test. Mandatory testing is costly and may be ineffective because it is not strictly a diagnostic tool.

A mandatory testing policy also carries certain moral, ethical, and legal implications. Some of these implications are reflected in the following questions, which each religious community or diocese should answer:

- Can the applicant be assured of absolute confidentiality if the results are positive?
- If confidentiality cannot be assured, is the order or diocese prepared to deal with the ethical and legal ramifications of revealing that the applicant is HIV positive? (HIV-positive persons may be subject to discrimination; loss of jobs, insurance, and friends; and alienation from family. Some have also committed suicide.)
- Does being HIV positive mean automatic denial of admission, or is such information considered in the overall profile of information that is gathered in determining acceptance or denial?
- Is the religious order or diocese prepared to assist the HIV-positive person to seek counselling and medical assistance to cope with the knowledge of having the virus.

If testing is mandatory, then these questions must be answered. There may be ongoing obligations to the applicant that cannot be denied, such as making available various resources for counselling and care. Many of these obligations are rooted in the essence of religious and Church community life.

In addition to questions regarding the testing of applicants, there are issues involving those who have been accepted and thus, are candidates, temporary professed, vowed, or ordained religious or clergy. Again, similar questions must be considered:

- Should candidates for religious life, temporary professed, or candidates for ordination be tested? (The same questions that apply to applicants also apply to these groups.)
- What are the obligations to the candidates, temporary professed, or seminarians about to be ordained if they acquire AIDS or ARC?

Concerning the temporary professed, one could refer to Canon 689 of the *Code of Canon Law*,[1] which has regulations governing those who acquire serious illnesses during this period. It is entirely possible that the person acquired the illness before his decision to enter a religious institute or seminary.

AIDS/ARC does not present a simple solution for the person who is not professed or ordained. If asked to leave, a person with AIDS/ARC may not be able to obtain or retain a job, health insurance, or housing because of the illness. Therefore, what are the overall obligations to ensure that financial support, healthcare, etc., will be available to the PWAs/PWARCs asked to leave? That the moral obligation may be as great as though the person were professed or ordained. In other words, the religious community or diocese may feel obliged to continue to support the individual.

In evaluating the best course to take, the major superior or bishop should consider the overall value of the person to the community or priesthood. How accepted is the person? How committed is the individual to religious life? How active and involved has the person been in the community? If AIDS or ARC had not been contracted, would the individual have been approved for temporary profession, final profession, or ordination?

Telling a person they are not suited for religious life or the priesthood is difficult enough and is usually done after much involved counselling. However, when AIDS compounds the issue, the diocese or religious community may have to deal with an ongoing obligation to the person and with other psychosocial and emotional sequelae. Leadership may also have to deal with the community concerning the decision to allow the person to stay or leave, particularly with regard to confidentiality issues. These factors are discussed later in this section.

PLANNING FOR CARE

Planning for the care of a PWA must involve the afflicted person as soon as possible. Usually a diagnosis of AIDS is made after a very serious illness. Therefore, in initial policy planning, a religious community or diocese may consider the development of a "core" support team to include the PWA, the local superior, the provincial, necessary medical professional, and others that may be identified by the PWA.

The primary goal of the support team is to assist the PWA in dealing with the many questions and issues that the illness brings. The PWA should plan for the time when he/she may no longer be able to make competent decisions. Have the wishes of the PWA been placed in writing and communicated to the superior or bishop?

Guidelines for the support team should be developed before the first case of AIDS appears. The role of each team member should be identified, as well as the issues and questions that each member should address.

SUPPORTIVE CARE ENVIRONMENT

What are the best ways to handle care and treatment of the religious PWA? Unfortunately, there may not be a "best" way, but focusing on the values of the Church and planning immediately for the eventuality are fundamental to any programs.

Once a diagnosis has been made, the primary concern should be for the person who is ill. The religious community or diocese should consider the following questions:[2]

- What provisions have been made for care?
- Is the religious order aware of which institutions provide the best care for PWAs?
- What provisions are needed to help the individual cope with the illness on an ongoing basis?
- Is the individual prepared to deal with revealing the illness to the community, the family, and the public?
- What resources are available within the civic community: outpatient facilities, mental health and social workers, and community-based organizations specifically formed to deal with AIDS issues?
- Can or should the individual remain within the local community or is another environment more appropriate because of care and support needs?
- Will the individual be able to continue ministry?

• Have the issues of durable power of attorney and living will been addressed and resolved?

Paramount in the care of PWAs is a supportive environment. The supportive environment should address physical, psychosocial, emotional, medical, spiritual, and ministry needs. The PWA will be dealing with an array of reactions, both positive and negative. Affected individuals will face emotions and feelings about themselves as well as the reactions of others, including members of the community or diocese, family, friends and co-workers.

In creating a supportive environment for the PWA, members of the religious community or diocese may become caregivers themselves. Caring for a terminally ill person can be physically and emotionally exhausting. Plans should include provisions for respite or relief for caregivers.

Later, other issues may surface:

• What planning is necessary for future care needs?
• Will hospice care be necessary?
• What is the extent of treatment desired in prolonging life?

RIGHT TO KNOW

The major superior or bishop has a need to know about the diagnosis, and the PWA/PWARC has the responsibility to inform the superior or bishop. The two of them then should work together to decide the best possible way to handle the situation. The affected individual should understand that secrecy may not be possible, for others may make assumptions or unavoidably obtain direct knowledge about the illness. The important issue is to protect the person's privacy as much as possible and to the extent the person desires. (Some PWAs/PWARCs are very open about their condition; others prefer to handle it alone.)

Should a religious community be told that a member has the condition? The decision to inform them must involve the PWA and his desire for privacy. Rather than leave it to speculation, the PWA should decide with the superior who should be told and how they should be told. Those who are informed will probably deal with the same feelings and emotions that the PWA experiences. Planning should address how best to support these individuals and answer their questions or concerns. It is important that these questions or concerns be addressed as honestly as possible, with a clear understanding of the PWA's wishes and a respect for confidentiality.

Fears about the illness may be minimized with education and preparation. Problems that may surface because of the perceived violation of vows also should be addressed. This calls for the religious and priests to look to their commitment to vowed life and their own vulnerability, to reach within and reflect on their call to serve others, and to reaffirm what it means to belong to their community and serve their brothers and sisters.

Ordained diocesan priests may not have the support system that a religious community offers; they may feel much more isolated. Bishops should be sensitive to this when counselling the priest and should assist in establishing a support system for him.

PWAs/PWARCs who are religious or clergy may delay seeking medical treatment because they fear being judged or condemned. As a result, they may die much sooner. This can be avoided if religious communities and dioceses develop sound policies and continuing educational programs and communicate this information to all members. These activities should not wait for the first case to surface.

INFORMING THE FAMILY

The PWA has the sole right to inform his/her family. It is not the right of the superior or bishop to do so without the PWA's knowledge and permission. Once this is done, family members will have many questions and concerns during the course of the illness. Some of the concerns may reflect their own inability to cope with their grief, anger, fears, and feelings. Therefore, regular communication with the informed family members is important. This communication should be established through mutual efforts of the PWA, the family, and the religious community or diocese.

AIDS AS MINISTRY

Women and men religious have long been in the forefront in meeting human needs. In such areas as healthcare, education, and missionary efforts, religious took an early lead. AIDS calls for similar pioneering efforts.

In speaking of religious; the Second Vatican Council states: "Christ should be shown contemplating on the mountain, announcing God's kingdom to the multitude, healing the sick and the maimed, turning sinners to conversion, blessing children, doing good to all and always obeying the will of the Father."[3] Thus AIDS, with all its pain, suffering, and stigma, provides religious an opportunity to minister to God's special people with all the hope of the Gospel. Jesus told us to touch and to heal. AIDS brings this call to some of the poorest and the most disenfranchised. It calls us to bring love and compassion to the alienated and the abandoned. It gives us an opportunity to use our resources in a ministry with many needs and challenges.

A NEED FOR SHARING

This section has raised many questions concerning AIDS within the Church community. Answers may vary among religious communities and dioceses; policies must be humane, caring, and compassionate. Confronting AIDS is not a time for judgment, recrimination, or undue concern about scandal; if there is a chance for scandal, it is not solely in the fact that vows may have been broken, but rather in how the issue is managed and how PWAs are treated, cared for, and cared about.

The cost of care for any one religious order could be devastating. Consideration may need to be given to regional care centers: religious orders and bishops could collaborate in establishing these centers and sharing the cost of care, even though they may not have anyone within their community or diocese with AIDS.

It is important for religious communities and dioceses to share their policies and educational programs. Equally important, they should share the issues, concerns, and questions that have surfaced and how they have responded. The best solutions will surface by working together rather than in isolation.

NOTES

1. *Code of Canon Law,* Latin-English Edition, Canon Law Society of America, Washington, DC, 1983, p. 263.
2. "A Proposed Policy of Assistance to Communities and Brothers of our Order Living with Acquired Immune Deficiency Syndrome," *AIDS Spector of Fear: Call for Concern, A Collection of Pastoral Responses,* CMI Journal, Vol 10, No. 10, August-September 1987.
3. Walter M. Abbott, *Constitution on the Church, Second Vatican Council,* American Press, New York, n. 46.

Ethical Guidelines for Healthcare Providers*

"You were darkness once, but now you are light in the Lord; be like children of light, for the effects of light are seen in complete goodness and right living and truth."

Eph 15:9

As mentioned earlier, Catholic doctrine and morality call and empower us to provide unqualified care to persons with AIDS (PWAs), their families, and their loved ones. The same sources also frame our moral obligation to apply resources toward preventing the spread of the deadly disease. However, as Catholic health institutions fulfill their mission to provide quality and compassionate healthcare in the face of the AIDS epidemic, they experience situations in which the application of Catholic moral principles seems unclear. When these situations arise, it helps to remember that AIDS is first and foremost a medical and public health problem. True, it has become the subject of intense public policy, regulatory, judicial, and ethical debate because of its highly infectious and fatal characteristics and the urgency associated with the epidemic; but because it is essentially a healthcare issue, the ethical questions AIDS poses are not fundamentally different from other ethical issues in healthcare.

This section is offered as a set of summary guidelines for use by administrators and health workers in the hospital, the long term care setting, and other places in the continuum of care. The guidelines may be

---

*By Diana Bader, OP, PhD, and Elizabeth McMillan, RSM, PhD. Earlier version published by The Catholic Health Association, St. Louis, MO, 1987.

helpful in responding to particular situations and in developing institutional policies and practices that are consistent with Catholic moral tradition as it applies to the AIDS epidemic.

CARE AND TREATMENT OF PATIENTS

The Patient's Perspective

1. Persons with AIDS and ARC deserve the same high standard of medical and nursing care as any other patient. The principle of *beneficence* requires that, as health professionals, we make reasonable efforts to further the good and well-being of all the persons for whom we care. Attitudes of discrimination, either overt or subtle, lead to a feeling of social isolation and are contrary to beneficence and to the fundamental moral virtues of compassion and justice that we owe to one another.

2. Because AIDS is inevitably fatal, questions about withholding or withdrawing treatment might seem different in this context than when faced in other treatment situations. Yet the principles that guide our decisions in other terminal illnesses will assist AIDS patients, their families, and health professionals to select appropriate treatment options.

In its *Statement on Euthanasia* (1980), the Vatican teaches that one is never obliged to use treatments that impose on the patient strain or suffering out of proportion to the benefits gained from using such techniques. It is, therefore, morally permissible to forego forms of treatment that would secure only a precarious and burdensome prolongation of life so long as the normal care due the sick person is not interrupted.

> It is also permissible to make do with the normal means that medicine can offer. Therefore, one cannot impose on anyone the obligation to have recourse to a technique which is already in use but which carries a risk or is burdensome. Such a refusal is not the equivalent of suicide; on the contrary, it should be considered as an acceptance of the human condition, or a wish to avoid the application of a medical procedure disproportionate to the results that can be expected, or a desire not to impose excessive expenses on the family or the Community.[1]

Although it is permissible to forego treatment that offers no benefit to the patient, it is important that treatment not be abandoned too soon, thus confirming for AIDS patients the hopelessness and despair of their situation. At all times, the goal is to provide for the comfort and well-being of the patient, including the effective management of pain.

3. Respect for individual *autonomy* requires that every effort be made to respect the wishes and decisions of the informed patient. PWAs usually will have decision-making capacity when their disease is diagnosed; however, the progression of the disease may involve eventual psychological or neurological impairment such that the patient may be unable to participate in treatment decisions. Therefore, it is advisable that steps be initiated as early as possible to identify and authorize a surrogate to make decisions when the patient is no longer able to decide for himself/herself. Such a surrogate decision maker may be a member of the immediate family or a close friend of the patient. Once such a person has been designated, the patient should discuss the choice with the attending physician, and the designation should be clearly documented in the patient's medical record.

4. Protecting the patient's right to privacy and confidentiality will require special efforts on the part of all those caring for AIDS patients.

Members of the healthcare team caring for the patient have a right to know the patient's diagnosis, but they are bound to the strictest standards of confidentiality regarding that information. This is true of information acquired regarding any patient, but it is especially relevant in diseases that carry a social stigma, such as sexually transmitted diseases. There may be pressure to release the information to unauthorized persons who, falsely, think that the presence of AIDS patients poses a significant risk and should be publicly disclosed.

The patient has the ultimate authority to control information regarding his/her diagnosis. In the absence of legal requirements, he/she is not obliged to disclose the diagnosis to anyone, including members of the immediate family. If there are particular circumstances that seem to override the patient's right to privacy, caregivers and counsellors should work sensitively with the patient to support him/her when deciding whether to disclose the information.

If the patient persists in refusing to disclose the information, the burden of proof rests on those who would act contrary to the patient's wishes. They would need to establish strong ethical justification based on anticipated harm to others because of failure to disclose. Such a situation may arise when a patient refuses to reveal to a spouse his/her condition, thus putting the spouse at risk of infection by continued sexual relations with the PWA.

Members of religious orders and the clergy have the same right to privacy and confidentiality regarding their medical diagnosis as any other patient.

Institutions have no obligation to make public disclosure regarding the AIDS diagnosis of employees or medical staff. However, they do have an obligation to protect patients. Administrators and supervisors, following good infection control policies, should, if at all possible, avoid assigning symptomatic persons with AIDS to areas where there may be an unusual risk of infection to patients by exchange of body fluids.

Because of the limited ways in which HIV is transmitted, good infection control policies and practices provide protection both for patients and employees.[2]

With regard to all these matters of patient privacy and confidentiality, the requirements of law will be a major consideration. Legal counsel should be consulted for advice.

The Healthcare Worker's Perspective

Healthcare workers who have the primary responsibility for a patient's well-being must provide high-quality, nonjudgmental care to their patients even at the risk of contracting a patient's disease. Physicians and nurses are charged by the ethics of their healing profession to treat patients with all forms of sickness and disease. It is inappropriate for any employee to compromise the treatment of patients with transmissible, lethal diseases such as AIDS on the grounds that such patients represent unacceptable medical risks.[3]

1. Although the high standards of the health professions require that all patients be treated fairly, humanely, and compassionately, health workers, being human, may react with discrimination, fear, stress, or hopelessness when asked to care for AIDS patients. Administrators and supervisors should be sensitive to these factors and should offer educational programs and counselling services to assist employees to overcome factors that impair their ability to provide consistent, humane care.

2. Certain life styles are usually associated with AIDS. The negative moral values attached to sexual promiscuity and intravenous drug use, for example, can translate into rejection of PWAs. No purpose is served by such moral recrimination. Moralizing only compounds the suffering of AIDS patients, diminishes the caregivers, and impedes the goals of unconditional and practical compassion.

Supervisors can help employees by providing the resources for their education and by helping them to identify phobic attitudes that may underlie discriminatory behavior. This should be provided through a coordinated and comprehensive education program for all employees.

3. The presence of a person with AIDS may evoke fear because of the perceived risk to life and health. Even when solid and convincing data indicate that risk of infection is minimal or nonexistent, health workers often are unpersuaded. This reminds us that reactions are shaped psychologically on a number of levels. Fear may arise not only from the perception of personal risk and phobic attitudes, but also from the hopelessness of the illness and the experience of witnessing the deaths of young patients in the prime of their adulthood. These factors may trigger emotions that override logic.

4. Because AIDS patients are very ill and require intense medical attention and vigorous emotional support, caregivers are susceptible to considerable stress. Stress may be manifested not only in physical and emotional "burnout" but also in negative behavior toward patients and co-workers. Administrators and supervisors have a moral obligation to provide the necessary professional and personal support for the healthcare workers, to ensure adequate staffing, and to provide for rotation of schedules to afford relief for employees.

INSTITUTIONAL POLICIES

The principle of justice requires that we give to each person what is due and that we balance the rights and benefits to the individual with the interests of society. This means that institutions are called to develop clear, coherent, just policies that will help prevent the spread of AIDS and guide their institutional responsibility toward patients, employees, and others. In the context of AIDS, this raises the following issues regarding institutional policies.

Testing and Screening for HIV

1. The test for the HIV antibody was licensed in 1985 to screen the U.S. blood supply. The test has many false positive results among low-risk persons and must be interpreted with caution. Thus far there is no fully accurate test for mass screening that definitely indicates whether a person has the virus and is infectious.

2. Routine testing and screening of patients or employees is not in the individual or public interest, and the discriminatory impact outweighs the potential benefit from testing asymptomatic persons. The burden of proof for the necessity of HIV screening rests with those proposing the test.

3. Selected screening of symptomatic persons whose personal conduct poses risk to others may be desirable on a case-by-case basis. Hospitals with a large number of AIDS patients may consider it useful to test selected asymptomatic employees for exposure, but always on a voluntary basis. Where such testing is in the community interest, the employee should give voluntary consent, in writing, based on accurate information provided in the informed consent process.

Coercive testing is not ethically appropriate. When a patient in a high-risk group refuses to undergo the antibody test, health workers should treat the patient according to strict infection control procedures but should not refuse necessary treatment.

4. Persons with a confirmed positive HIV antibody test should be counselled and helped to understand the range of implications of the positive result.

Management of Information

1. The norms governing confidentiality apply in all matters related to AIDS. This is an area of particular tension, positioning the individual's interest in liberty and privacy against the public's interest in health and safety. For the individual, measures to control the spread of AIDS may invade privacy, constrain sexual conduct, and limit personal liberty. Tolerance of these results may be justified when harm to other individuals is at stake and the harm can be effectively removed or minimized by the disclosure of information. Expert legal advice is encouraged.

2. Cases of AIDS are reportable to the public health authorities everywhere in the United States. Because reporting requirements vary from state to state, the relevant state laws should be referred to in reporting. Aside from such legal requirements and the need to know that relates to providing treatment, healthcare professionals have a moral duty to keep confidential all facts about a patient's diagnosis and treatment.

3. Disclosure may be appropriate and obligatory to those unequivocally at risk (e.g., a patient's spouse or lover). Patients who are infected with HIV but who do not have AIDS should be encouraged to inform their contacts. If they refuse and continue their high-risk behavior, physicians

and hospitals may be justified in seeking the assistance of public health authorities to alert those at risk. In such cases, there is a strong moral warrant for disclosure because of the deadly nature of the disease and the serious risk to those involved. The obligation to disclose is greater where the level of risk is greater (e.g., frequent spousal sexual contact) or in communities where the infection is more prevalent and high-risk behavior is accepted.

Employment

1. Healthcare employees who have been diagnosed as HIV infected do not necessarily become unable to discharge their duties. Steps should not be taken to terminate such employees as long as they are able to perform their duties and the disease has not debilitated them.

2. The presence of a symptomatic PWA might create unnecessary risk to patients in areas where exchange of body fluids may occur (such as surgery). The employee might be reassigned to another area but should generally retain the status, salary, and benefits of the prior assignment.

3. Physicians, nurses, and other healthcare workers have no ethical obligation to inform administration, their supervisors, or their patients of their diagnosis unless their health status presents a disproportionate risk to patients. These persons enjoy the same right of privacy and confidentiality as any other PWA.

4. Although it is recommended that employers not *require* HIV antibody testing of employees in high-risk groups, it may be proper to encourage an employee suspected of HIV infection to be tested so that treatment can begin and the effects of the infection can be minimized.

5. In all areas of AIDS-related employment decisions, expert legal advice should be sought.

Preventing the Spread of AIDS

As long as there remains no vaccine against HIV and no cure for AIDS and ARC, the sole means of prevention is the creation of a well-informed public who will take the necessary precautions to prevent the spread of the virus.

Administrators should help to provide the following for their employees, patients, and community:

1. Information about the nature of the disease, the ways it is spread, the populations at risk, and its seriousness as a public health problem. In

this regard, the U.S. Surgeon General's report on AIDS should be read by all persons involved in healthcare and by those involved in the education of others within the institution and in the community.

2. Education about the moral aspects of conduct that creates risk for AIDS. Elements of this moral framework include:

- Traditional Catholic teachings supporting stable, faithful, monogamous marriages as the appropriate locus for sexual relationships.
- A sense of personal dignity and self-esteem that enables individuals to relate to others without relying on sexual intercourse as the primary means of communication within a relationship.
- Efforts to restore to genital sexual acts their meaning as a form of communication expressing serious, long-term commitment between the parties.
- Appreciation that even those who do not share these values have a social obligation to prevent the spread of AIDS by avoiding high-risk behavior.

3. Recognition that ours is a pluralistic society and that not all persons will be able or willing to change their behavior. For these reasons, according to the U.S. bishops' statement on AIDS,

[E]ducational efforts, if grounded in the broader moral vision outlined [earlier in the statement], could include accurate information about prophylactic devices or other practices proposed by some medical experts as potential means of preventing AIDS. We are not promoting the use of prophylactics, but merely providing information that is part of the factual picture. Such a factual presentation should indicate that abstinence outside of marriage and fidelity within marriage as well as the avoidance of intravenous drug abuse are the only morally correct and medically sure ways to prevent the spread of AIDS.[4]

Research and Experimentation

The primary goal of medical research is to promote the development of general scientific knowledge about disease. The primary goal of clinical therapy is to benefit the individual patient. When medical research is conducted in the clinical therapy setting (e.g., the testing of new drugs, vaccines, or diagnostic measures), the goals of research and treatment may become confused and the competing interests of parties involved in AIDS research and those providing treatment may become a critical issue. This may be especially true when new and unvalidated therapies are being tested on AIDS patients. PWAs are members of a special population with a fatal condition who may be willing to incur greater risk to themselves in an attempt to prolong their own lives or in order to serve the good of others.

The following guidelines should apply to the conduct of AIDS research in Catholic institutions:

1. The research should be conducted by competent investigators, following a design that will yield clinically reliable results.
2. The local institutional review board should review and monitor all AIDS-related research and experimentation to ensure that all acceptable legal and ethical norms are met.
3. Patients should be protected from disproportionate risks; a careful risk/benefit balance is required for approval of an experimental protocol.
4. Careful attention should be given to the protection of the PWA's rights in the matters of informed consent, privacy, and the selection of subjects for research.
5. Because of the danger of coercion or duress with AIDS patients, who may feel desperate for some form of therapy, special protections should be developed to ensure that therapies are not used until they have been tested and verified according to accepted procedures for standard clinical trials.
6. Provision should be made for compensation for injury induced through research and should be clearly stated in informed consent documents.
7. Competent legal advice should be sought when establishing all such policies.

CORPORATE RELATIONS AND SOCIAL POLICY

Framework for Ministry: Charity, Truth, and Justice

The preceding discussion of the ethical issues makes it clear that health professionals have a professional obligation to respond. Furthermore, the epidemic proportions of AIDS expand this obligation into the broader context of public health and safety.

The mission of Catholic healthcare revolves around the core values of truth, charity, and justice. The AIDS epidemic offers Catholic institutions a unique opportunity to show the community what we understand by these words. A commitment to *truth* requires that our institutions communicate fully and clearly the medical and epidemiological facts of the disease in a context that also includes the human and moral aspects of AIDS in social relationships. The message should educate people about how to avoid AIDS by avoiding risky behavior and at the same time help them to avoid "AFRAIDS" (acute fear regarding AIDS). *Charity* requires that we work together to overcome our own fears about AIDS and assist people in need. *Justice* calls for a special sensitivity to the fact that high-risk groups may be less likely to receive public sympathy because of many persons' misguided notions of moral righteousness.

Corporate Relations: The Institution's Posture Toward the Community

Charity: refusing none; linking with others to respond. One test of the institution's credibility in the community is to listen to the people who live and work there, especially to those who are developing local AIDS programs. Do they speak of the facility as being informed, competent, and ready to care well for people with AIDS? A facility with a pattern of referring AIDS patients to other facilities should begin to prepare its own staff to admit them.

Reluctance to accept AIDS patients who cannot pay for care belies the mission we claim. Catholic hospitals and long term care facilities should take the lead in organizing the healthcare community to share the financial burden of caring for uninsured PWAs. Our posture should be proactive in putting together a response.

Long term care facilities have special challenges because they are residential facilities and may not be staffed to respond with the kind of care AIDS patients need. They cannot, however, excuse themselves from beginning to address this major gap in the continuum of care. The Catholic tradition suggests that the need should be met by a number of facilities working in concert.

In communities hit early by AIDS, well-organized groups of trained volunteers offer a range of direct services to PWAs. Hospitals and nursing homes should be building links with these groups to develop similar programs where they are nonexistent or only beginning. Hospice and home care programs should also be working to offer comprehensive support.

Truth: responsibility without panic. Healthcare facilities, especially hospitals, have resources, credibility, and status in the community. This fact places a special burden on those facilities in educating the public about AIDS. Through publications, media opportunities, public service announcements, and other resources, healthcare has a forum not available to many educational institutions and religious groups.

It is important, therefore, that Catholic healthcare communicate the ethical, medical, and epidemiological facts about AIDS. We should speak out on issues of health and public safety in terms of respectful human relationships (both in society at large and in intimate sexual relationships). With effective messages about AIDS transmission, we can help people evaluate their sexual practices in light of Gospel and Church teaching and respect for their own bodies and those of their partners. Likewise, although clear and correct information about AIDS transmission should help to allay public fears about contracting AIDS by casual contact, information alone may not always suffice. It may be necessary, for example, to counter talk of quarantines for PWAs by speaking out to support the rights of these people.

As discussed earlier, it is equally important that representatives of Catholic healthcare use the opportunities afforded them to correct the idea that AIDS is punishment for sinful behavior. Such an attitude, personally demeaning to the person with AIDS, has the further effect of isolating the sick person most in need of community support. It is all the more urgent that these ethical points be made forcefully by a Catholic voice because some persons both within and outside the Church think that Catholic moral teaching sanctions a kind of retribution theology.

Social Policy: The Institutional Role in Shaping Public Policy

Justice: promoting public health without jeopardizing the dignity of individuals. The obligation of a healthcare institution to comply with the laws and regulations governing its activity becomes even more important in the face of the AIDS epidemic. Compliance is never a simple matter, even in ordinary times; it is all the more difficult in the case of AIDS. Not only are the epidemiological data difficult to keep up with and the staff anxieties difficult to manage, but the challenge is compounded because patterns of transmission in the United States are linked to groups who have historically suffered discrimination in our society.

Reporting cases of AIDS to public health authorities may raise few ethical problems, but a requirement to report all HIV-positive test results is more problematic. Justifications for reporting test results are tied to health planning: measuring the scope of the problem to project services and costs, developing strategies for financing care, and educating the public to prevent the spread of the disease. Institutions can provide useful data for health planning purposes in statistical, aggregate form while protecting the privacy of those whose tests are being reported. Those who manage patient records should make certain that internal processes for gathering data ensure the anonymity of the data as it leaves the institution.

Some public health officials have called for routine screening of certain segments of the population. For example, some have recommended that AIDS screening be done routinely at all prenatal, family planning, drug abuse, and sexually transmitted disease clinics. Their concerns go beyond merely tracking the disease; they are attempting to intervene in the lives of these people for curative and preventive purposes. Using the test diagnostically, however, offers only limited possibilities for therapeutic intervention, and most experts agree that widespread testing would cost far more than it would be worth in terms of the actual usefulness of the information collected.

Numerous ethical issues, discussed earlier in this section, should be raised by institutions or clinics that would consider participating in selective screening programs. Not only may the privacy of the individual be at stake, but public trust in healthcare institutions may be threatened as well. Further care should be taken not to undermine social relationships already severely strained by the threat of AIDS.

All these ethical concerns are placed in sharp relief by the special question of contact tracing: systematically attempting to discover the sexual partners of someone who has been found to be HIV positive. Because such programs require the collection of person-specific information, we should help to shape a public policy that protects confidentiality and prohibits discrimination. We should also insist that adequate counselling be made an integral feature of the program.

A particularly sensitive area is insurance coverage for people in high-risk groups. Is it appropriate to refuse coverage to an individual solely because he/she is a member of a high-risk group? Should insurance companies be permitted to exclude individuals from coverage on the basis of a positive HIV test? Several states have made it illegal to use an HIV test as a criterion of insurability. Although insurance companies understandably may take a conservative posture in light of future uncertainties about the scope of the AIDS epidemic, they should be expected to carry a fair share of the risk. Catholic providers, particularly those who have equity in insurance companies and managed care entities, should play a leadership role in making sure that coverage is just.

MISSION AND REEVALUATION

In all these questions related to the AIDS epidemic, the measure of our actions is the gospel mission we have been given. We need to be sensitive to the fact that AIDS calls for a reevaluation of our habitual ways of caring for patients, relating to the community, and acting in the larger political and social arena. This reevaluation in turn may require a reordering of professional and institutional relationships as we attempt to give a clearer witness to this mission in the healthcare ministry.

NOTES

1. "Declaration on Euthanasia," Sacred Congregation for Doctrine of the Faith, May 5, 1980.
2. See *Morbidity and Mortality Weekly Report*, Centers for Disease Control, Vol. 34, no. 45, August 21, 1987.
3. "Position Paper: Acquired Immunodeficiency Syndrome," Health and Public Policy Committee, American College of Physicians and the Infectious Diseases Society of America. *Annals of Internal Medicine*, Vol. 104, 1986, pp. 575-581.
4. United States Catholic Conference Administrative Board, "The Many Faces of AIDS: A Gospel Response," *Origins*, Dec. 24, 1987, p. 486.

Legal Implications for Healthcare Providers*

"But surely the Law does not allow us to pass judgment on a man without giving him a hearing and discovering what he is about?"

Jn 7:51

The AIDS epidemic has affected U.S. healthcare providers in a way unprecedented in this century. The psychosocial ramifications of this disease and the pervasive anxiety that it produces have touched every aspect of healthcare. Healthcare providers and consumers, as well as families and friends of healthcare providers, have increasingly been forced to deal with their anxieties about this condition. No healthcare provider or institution in the United States can avoid these issues in the future.

One survey revealed that 37 percent of a sample study of the general population feared contracting AIDS in a general acute care hospital that treats AIDS patients. Despite a century of progress in life-saving medical technology, our institutions of wellness have now come to be perceived by many as institutions of doom and death.[1]

Although the law does not have a uniform response to this disease, many jurisdictions have enacted legislation reflecting various societal responses to the epidemic. Also, recent court decisions on AIDS issues have pointed the way to a clearer understanding of individual rights and responsibilities. Finally, the law does provide general guidance for providers by analogy through longstanding legal principles. The most

*By Mark A. Kadzielski, JD. Earlier versions published by The Catholic Health Association, St. Louis, MO, 1987, and *Health Progress,* May 1986.

significant principles are those of privacy and confidentiality and of fairness and antidiscrimination in employment.

CONFIDENTIALITY AND PRIVACY ISSUES

Confidentiality principles in the healthcare setting are contained in many laws and regulations throughout the United States. Essentially, these principles focus on the right of any individual to have his/her health matters treated privately and without unauthorized disclosure to those who have no need to know such information, including other patients and healthcare workers not involved in providing direct care to that person. In many jurisdictions, disclosure of confidential patient information is both a crime and a tort, giving rise to both fines and civil damages.[2] The general rationale for such confidentiality, of course, is the notion that every individual has a right to privacy regarding personal healthcare and has a right to determine who has access to such information.

Confidentiality issues in the context of AIDS have appeared to conflict with public health concerns. Few dispute the appropriateness of public health reporting of confirmed cases of infectious diseases, including AIDS. But some have argued that all patients in health facilities should be tested for HIV exposure and that the results should be disseminated so that individuals in the healthcare institution can be assured of their personal health safety. Others have argued that all prospective and current healthcare employees should be tested for HIV antibodies to determine whether they should be permitted to work in healthcare. The advisability of such suggestions are discussed later, but it is important to remember that they concern an individual's basic right to privacy.[3]

Patients' rights to privacy and confidentiality, sometimes overlooked in the healthcare setting, cannot be selectively violated depending on the disease in question. For patients and employees diagnosed as having AIDS, confidentiality and privacy considerations should still apply. Dissemination of confidential patient information to those who have no legal or rational requirement to know it may result in the healthcare provider's criminal and/or civil liability. Given the highly charged psychosocial atmosphere surrounding this syndrome, the imposition of such liability in an appropriate case is not unlikely.

The advent of the HIV blood test has made this situation more critical. In March 1985 the federal Food and Drug Administration licensed the HIV blood test to detect antibodies to the AIDS virus. The federal government authorized the establishment of alternative testing sites for HIV testing where individuals who wished to determine their antibody status could do so anonymously and free of charge. Blood banks and plasma centers applied this test to all blood donated for human use in order to safeguard the U.S. blood supply.[4] The availability of the test to the medical community, however, brings new pressures to bear on the privacy and confidentiality rights of patients and employees.

The state of medical information on this test, however, is constantly developing. According to current medical knowledge, AIDS itself is only one end of the HIV spectrum. That is, it is possible to have HIV antibodies without any other evidence of the condition and to remain asymptomatic, possibly indefinitely. It is also possible to have some signs and symptoms of disease, which may abate after a time, to develop AIDS-related complex or full-blown AIDS.[5]

For these reasons, it is not clear what a positive test for HIV antibodies would demonstrate other than that the person had been infected by the virus at some point in the past. The test does not indicate that the individual currently has AIDS, will develop ARC, or will develop AIDS, and the test itself is not diagnostic. Unlike other medical tests for infectious diseases, this test alone cannot detect AIDS, and it is also possible to have false positive and false negative test results.[6]

What HIV test results mean in any predictive way is therefore unknown at present. Given the fact that the test results are not predictive, it appears difficult to justify, either legally or logically, the blanket screening of patients or employees in the healthcare setting. Neither the Centers for Disease Control (CDC) nor the American Hospital Association (AHA) recommends such screening.[7]

Recent CDC recommendations for the prevention of HIV transmission in healthcare facilities focus on universal precautions for handling blood and body fluids of all patients. These recommendations emphasize the need for a consensual discussion before HIV testing in the healthcare setting. The CDC recommends that "when deemed appropriate, testing of individual patients may be performed on agreement between the patient and the physician." In addition, for more wide-scale testing programs, the CDC recommends obtaining the person's consent and ensuring that "confidentiality safeguards are in place to limit knowledge of test results to those directly involved in care of infected patients or as required by law." The AHA similarly has recently recommended obtaining consent from patients before testing, noting that, because "a positive HIV test can have profound implications for an individual's health and lifestyle, it is widely accepted that patients should receive information about the implications of HIV testing before and after the test is performed."[8]

Practical implications of the suggestion that everyone be tested for AIDS antibodies must also be considered. Recent reports indicate that, at least 1,000,000 persons in the United States alone have been exposed to HIV.[9] The nondefinitive nature of HIV test results begs the question: "What do you do with the test results once you have them?" The answer, of course, may involved unjustified discrimination against the tested persons. Given the risks to individual privacy and confidentiality such required testing creates, and the lack of clear-cut benefits, widespread mandatory screening with the tests currently available is inadvisable at this point.

As noted, the CDC has recommended that healthcare workers not be screened for HIV antibodies. Moreover, several states, most notably California, Florida, and Wisconsin, have enacted legislation that requires heightened confidentiality regarding anyone subjected to the HIV test.[10] California requires prior written consent for the test and punishes unauthorized disclosure of HIV test results by both criminal and civil penalties. California also prohibits the use of test results for purposes of insurability or suitability for employment. Such legislation, which has been and will be considered in similar formats in other states, attempts to balance the privacy and public health concerns.

PERSONNEL ISSUES

The problems of how to deal with healthcare personnel who either have been exposed to the virus or fear exposure to the virus in their work environment are neither simple nor specifically addressed under the law. Several significant issues, however, warrant discussion.[11]

Physical Handicap Discrimination

Although the issue is not completely settled, it appears that HIV infection, including AIDS, is a physical handicap under state and federal law.[12] Other physical conditions such as high blood pressure, diabetes, and tuberculosis have been held to be physical handicaps under such laws.[13]

It is reasonable to treat all employees with HIV infection as entitled to all the legal protections afforded other handicapped individuals. Accordingly, applying principles of handicap discrimination law to this situation, a healthcare institution may not terminate or otherwise discriminate against an employee with HIV infection unless (1) the employee cannot, even with reasonable accommodation, perform the essential elements of the job, or (2) the employee cannot perform the job without causing a present and substantial danger to the health and safety of the employee or others.[14]

Regarding the possibility that HIV-infected employees could catch opportunistic diseases from patients they are treating, the CDC does not believe that the danger is significant as long as standard infection control procedures are utilized. However, the CDC does recommend that the healthcare organization, in conjunction with the employee's physician, evaluate each infected employee periodically on a case-by-case basis to determine the danger of contracting such diseases from patients.[15] In addition, HIV-infected employees should be examined to determine whether they are a danger to their own or others' health and safety. Current information indicates that, if proper infection control precautions are taken, such a danger would probably not exist, but health facilities should be sure to use the most current medical information regarding AIDS in assessing infected employees.

Tort Liability to Patients and Employees

Theoretically, healthcare facilities are subject to tort liability to patients and/or employees who might contract HIV infection, including AIDS, as a result of exposure to an HIV-infected employee. However, given current knowledge about how the virus is transmitted, the danger of liability appears remote. To prevail on such a theory, the patient or employee would have to prove that the healthcare organization violated its duty of care by allowing such an employee to continue working. As long as a health facility takes the precautions recommended in the most current medical literature, the chances of tort liability should be greatly minimized.

Workers' Compensation

If an employee does develop AIDS or become infected by HIV as the result of on-the-job exposure, the employee will undoubtedly be eligible for state workers' compensation benefits. But if the CDC guidelines on AIDS in the healthcare workplace are followed, the chance of an employer incurring workers' compensation liability in this fashion is remote. A more likely source of liability is HIV-infected employees who contract opportunistic infections from patients they are treating. Workers' compensation and antidiscrimination employment laws generally prohibit an employer from refusing to hire or retain an employee simply because of the risk of potential workers' compensation liability.[16] In addition, if all proper precautions for preventing the spread of infectious disease have been taken, the healthcare employer may be permitted to defend against such a compensation claim on the ground that the employee contracted the opportunistic disease because of a preexisting condition unrelated to the workplace.

OSHA and Wrongful Termination Liability

State and federal Occupational Safety and Health Administration (OSHA) laws give employees the right to a safe working environment and prohibit employers from disciplining employees who assert that right. Under such health and safety laws, an employee may lawfully refuse to work in proven unsafe conditions and may also insist on wearing safety equipment while working.[17] In the context of AIDS, this means that an employee may lawfully refuse to treat an HIV-infected patient if doing so is unsafe. However, since the virus is known to be transmitted only through the exchange of body fluids, it appears that caring for HIV-infected patients is not inherently unsafe. Moreover, if healthcare providers take reasonable precautions such as those recommended by the CDC, the treatment of HIV-infected patients, including AIDS patients, should not pose a health threat. In general, therefore, an employee who refuses to treat such patients may lawfully be disciplined for insubordination.

When an employee insists on wearing more protective gear (masks, gloves, etc.) than the healthcare facility thinks necessary, the employer should investigate the employee's rationale and conduct appropriate in-service education on the transmissibility of this disease. Some states forbid discrimination against employees for complaining about health hazards, even if there is no actual danger, as long as the employee has a reasonable belief that such a danger exists.[18] For example, in a case before the California Labor Commissioner, several nurses claimed they had been unlawfully transferred because of their insistence on wearing masks and other protective gear thought to be unnecessary by the hospital.[19] Although the hearing officer dismissed their complaints because he concluded that the transfers were not related to their insistence on wearing the gear, he noted that the nurses' concern was "understandable" and that their conduct was protected under California labor laws.

In addition, at least one California court has held that disciplining an employee for complaining about a health hazard, even if a hazard did not actually exist, may constitute "wrongful termination" against public policy and subject the employer to liability for compensatory and punitive damages.[20] Thus, employers who discipline employees for insisting on more-than-reasonable precautions or for complaining about the danger of treating HIV-infected patients, including AIDS patients, risk liability under state and federal OSHA statutes as well as under common law wrongful termination theories.

COMBATTING EMPLOYEES' FEARS

Healthcare providers should adopt and enforce infection control policies based on the most recent medical information to prevent the spread of this disease and its attendant anxiety throughout health facilities. (Sample policies are found in the Appendix.) In-service educational programs on patient confidentiality and privacy rights, as well as on the other legal rights of patients and employees, can also reassure healthcare workers by presenting accurate information about the risks they face.

NOTES

1. H. Anderson, "37% Fear Contracting AIDS in Hospital," *Modern Healthcare*, Nov. 8, 1985, p. 28; an AMA-sponsored poll found that 48% of American adults believe that it is "very likely" that AIDS will eventually kill "a large share" of the U.S. population, *AIDS Policy & Law*, Oct. 21, 1987.
2. *Hospital Law Manual*, Medical Records. Section 3 (1983). For example, the California Confidentiality of Medical Information Act, Civil Code Section 56 *et seq.*, punishes unauthorized disclosure of confidential medical information as a misdemeanor and imposes civil liability in the form of compensatory damages for all

disclosure-related economic loss or personal injury, punitive damages not to exceed $3,000, attorneys' fees not to exceed $1,000, and the costs of litigation. Tort remedies generally available to patients whose healthcare information is wrongfully disclosed include defamation, intentional and negligent infliction of emotional distress, and invasion of privacy.

3. U.S. Constitution, Fourth Amendment; Cal. Const. Article 1 § 1; Antieu, *Modern Constitutional Law,* Chapter 2: Society's Interest in the Privacy of the Individual.

4. "Provisional Public Health Service Inter-Agency Recommendations for Screening Donated Blood and Plasma for Antibody to the Virus Causing AIDS," 34 *CDC Morbidity and Mortality Weekly Report,* Jan. 11, 1985, pp. 1-5.

5. "Progress on AIDS," 15 U.S. Department of Health and Human Services, *FDA Drug Bulletin* 29, Oct. 1985.

6. S. H. Weiss, "Screening Test for HTLV-III (AIDS Agent) Antibodies: Specificity, Sensitivity, and Applications," *Journal of the American Medical Association* 253, Jan. 11, 1985, pp. 221-225.

7. "Recommendations for Preventing Transmission of Infection with Human T-Lymphotropic Virus III/Lymphadenopathy-Associated Virus in the Workplace," 34 *CDC Morbidity and Mortality Weekly Report* 682, Nov. 15, 1985; AHA, "Management of HTLV-III/LAV Infection in the Hospital," Jan. 1986. A recent case, *Glover v. Eastern Nebraska Community Office of Retardation,* 56 U.S.L.W. 2560 (D. Neb. April 12, 1988), struck down a mandatory HIV antibody testing program for staff members at a Nebraska facility for the mentally retarded. The court held that the mandatory testing was an unconstitutional infringement on these healthcare workers' rights to be free from unreasonable searches and seizures under the Fourth Amendment.

8. "Recommendations for Prevention of HIV Transmission in Health-Care Settings," 36 *CDC Morbidity and Mortality Weekly Report,* no. 2S, at 14S-15S, Aug. 21, 1987; American Hospital Association Policy Statement, Nov. 19, 1987; "Physician Use of the HIV Antibody Test: The Need for Consent, Counseling, Confidentiality and Caution," *Journal of the American Medical Association* 259, Jan. 8, 1988, pp. 264-265.

9. M. Krim, "AIDS: The Challenge to Science and Medicine," 15 *Hastings Center Report* 2, Aug. 1985; *AIDS Policy & Law,* Aug. 12, 1987.

10. California Health and Safety Code § 199.20 *et seq.* (1985); § 381.606 Florida Statutes (1985); Wisconsin Statutes § 103.15, § 146.023, § 146.025, § 619.12, and § 631.90 (1985).

11. Facilities may also face problems under collective bargaining agreements as well as under the National Labor Relations Act governing "concerted activity" by employees.

12. Discrimination against the handicapped is governed by the federal Vocational Rehabilitation Act of 1973, 29 U.S.C.A. § 794 (1985) as well as by state laws. The scope of the federal law is limited to recipients of federal financial assistance and is the subject of much controversy. In one federal district court to date, AIDS has been held to be a physical handicap under federal law. *Thomas v. Atascadero Unified School District,* 662 F. Supp. 376 (C.D. Cal. 1987). The Thomas case involved a child with AIDS who was barred from kindergarten by the school district after he bit a classmate. In ordering reinstatement pursuant to Section 504 of the federal Vocational Rehabilitation Act of 1973, federal District Judge Alicemarie Stotler held that AIDS was a protected handicap under the terms of that statute. More recently,

the Ninth Circuit Court of Appeals ordered a teacher with AIDS reinstated under this same authority. *Chalk v. U.S. District Court*, 832 F.2d 1158 (9th Cir. 1987), further opinion at 840 F.2d 701 (9th Cir. 1988).

13. *American National Insurance Co. v. Calif. Fair Employment and Housing Commission*, 32 Cal. 3d 603 (1982) [high blood pressure]; *Bentivegna v. United States Department of Labor*, 694 F.2d 609, 621 (9th Cir. 1982) [diabetes]; and *Arline v. School Board of Nassau County*, 107 S.Ct. 1123 (1987) [tuberculosis]. Although the *Arline* case did not directly address AIDS and HIV infection, recent legislation leaves little doubt that they are protected handicaps. S.557, the Civil Rights Restoration Act of 1987, that became law after a congressional override on March 22, 1988 of President Reagan's veto, codified the *Arline* principles that persons with any 'contagious disease or infection' are protected under Section 504 of the federal Vocational Rehabilitation Act.

14. California Gov't. Code § 12940 (a) (1985). This analysis assumes that HIV infection, including AIDS, will be held to a physical handicap in *Calif. Department of Fair Employment and Housing v. Raytheon Co.*, FEP 83-84 L1-0310p L-33998 (1986), judicial appeal pending in Santa Barbara Superior Court (1988). Several municipalities in California to date (e.g. Los Angeles, Berkeley, West Hollywood and San Francisco) and the County of Santa Clara have enacted broad AIDS antidiscrimination ordinances, as has the District of Columbia, and the adoption of other local ordinances on this subject is anticipated.

15. *See* notes 7 and 8.

16. *See, e.g.*, Calif. Labor Code § 3200 *et seq.*; *Sterling Transit Co. v. California Fair Employment Practice Commission*, 121 Cal.App.3d 791, 799-800 (1981).

17. 29 U.S.C. § 660(c); Cal. Labor Code § 6310. Although the federal OSHA law creates an exclusive remedy through the federal Department of Labor, many state OSHA laws permit a private right of action in addition to adjudication by a state agency. The federal Occupational Safety and Health Administration is planning to enforce the CDC guidelines and recommendations pursuant to a Joint Advisory Notice issued by the Departments of Labor and Health and Human Services, 52 Fed. Reg. 41818 (Oct. 30, 1987). OSHA will respond to employee complaints and conduct inspections to ensure that these CDC guidelines are being followed. OSHA also plans to formulate more specific regulations to provide further guidance regarding its investigation and enforcement functions regarding such diseases as AIDS.

18. California Labor Code §§ 6310-6311; *Hentzel v. Singer Co.*, 138 Cal.App.3d 290, 299 (1982).

19. *Bernales et al. v. San Francisco Dept. of Public Health*, Nos. 11-17001-1 through 4 (Cal. Labor Commissioner, Sept. 9, 1985).

20. *Hentzel v. Singer*, 138 Cal.App.3d at 299.

9

Summary and Conclusion: The Catholic Response

"Master, why was this man born blind? Was it because of his own sin or those of his parents?" "Neither," Jesus answered, "but to demonstrate the power of God"
Jn 9:11-3

Jesus thus reached out to heal the blind man. As Catholics and Christians, we must reject the concept that AIDS, or any illness, is punishment for sin. We must reach out with a healing touch.[1] "Rather than God's retribution, suffering becomes an occasion for God's love and compassion to be demonstrated. Where people of faith reach out and touch those with AIDS, they can transform suffering into a living example of God's compassionate love."[2]

AIDS is going to be with us for a long time. The future for persons with AIDS (PWAs) or AIDS-related complex (PWARCs) appears to be bleak, but it can be hopeful. The challenges seem almost overwhelming, but each challenge presents an opportunity for us not only to witness to the Gospel, but to make it come "alive" throughout the world.

As Church and a community of faith, we are given the opportunity through the AIDS crisis to assist people in need.[3] As teacher, the Church can educate and create an understanding of how God's unconditional compassion, love, and mercy are manifested in the pain and suffering of PWAs. As a community of faith, we are responsible to God to seek out the truth and help overcome the panic, hysteria, pain of discrimination, and unjustices that have occurred because of AIDS. We should demonstrate the love and compassion of Jesus in accepting and caring for PWAs/PWARCs. We can be a resource to society in overcoming fear, bigotry, and discrimination.

The Catholic Church is an active and vital resource throughout the world. Our faith, based on the Gospel of Jesus, is the most valued resource that we possess in addressing the multiplicity of issues surrounding AIDS. To mobilize and overcome the AIDS tragedy, we must demonstrate the compassionate love of Jesus in educating people and assisting them to overcome their biases. These biases thwart the efforts of all to work together to solve the problem, develop programs, and care for those suffering from AIDS.

To educate others, we must demonstrate our belief in the Gospel tradition by overcoming our own biases and negative attitudes. We cannot be judgmental and hateful. We must be true witnesses to the Gospel of Jesus. We can shape the world's response to AIDS and to persons with AIDS. As Church, we must demonstrate universally our commitment and conviction.

GUIDELINES FOR ADDRESSING AIDS

An overwhelming task lies before us. To confront it, we must exercise leadership and ask: How can we as Church use our resources and influence in addressing the AIDS tragedy?[4]

- Every bishop, priest, and religious should address his or her personal attitude about AIDS and become educated regarding its implications for society.

- Every parish should reaffirm the Church's principles on moral conduct. At the same time, the Church will not tolerate bigotry and discrimination against homosexuals, IV drug abusers, and others who are afflicted.

- Every religious and layperson should realize that they have a role in addressing AIDS issues. They, too, should understand AIDS and its implications for society. To help in meeting the needs, they must understand that everyone in the Church and society at large must work toward committing the necessary resources to accomplish these ends.

- The Church cannot work alone in addressing the crisis. Although every bishop, priest, religious, and layperson should understand their personal role, they should also work with others to ensure a comprehensive plan to resolving the problems as quickly as possible.

- The Church should work with government and the private sector to make certain that funding is available for research and treatment and that those who cannot afford care can more easily gain access to it. The Church should advocate for needed changes in public policy and should be a leader in educating the public regarding the necessary policy changes.
- Catholic healthcare facilities and organizations should mobilize in their communities to create coalitions or to become members of existing ones to ensure that all the problems are being addressed.
- Every person should be encouraged to read the Surgeon General's report.
- Health and social service organizations should share resources. For example, if no nursing home is available for the care of PWAs, several facilities perhaps can unite to develop and operate one. Working together we can create alternative housing, financial assistance programs, and other services. Parish convents, vacant schools, motherhouses, etc., all have the potential to be used for alternative care or resource centers to meet needs.
- As previously indicated, the gay communities in most locales were the first to organize to meet the needs of PWAs. They are a valuable resource and should be asked to play a vital role in planning for services and programs.
- The needs of minority groups are great and have largely been overlooked. The IV drug abusers that have AIDS are primarily from the black and Hispanic population. Many do not have access to healthcare services. They are usually poor and have low self-esteem. They tend to be transient, so it is difficult to educate them about AIDS and to get them to change their life style. The Church has an important call here: by working with black and Hispanic leaders, programs can be developed to meet the serious needs of these populations.
- The family is the core of society, and AIDS presents a special threat to family harmony. Parents may be overwhelmed to learn that their child is an IV drug abuser or homosexual. They often learn this when visiting their son or daughter in a hospital far from home, and they often find they must cope with the news alone. What happens when they return home; whom do they tell? Who will console them?

These issues present a serious need for pastoral care and social service counselling. Healing must take place, guilt must be alleviated, and blame must be laid to rest. Both the family and the PWA should understand what they are facing. They need to feel love and concern for each other.

The Church can play an important role in resolving these conflicts and bringing about healing. Every community should have pastoral care and social service programs sponsored by the Church to meet these special needs. If they cannot develop their own, then they should network with others who have them. These networks can also serve in the continuity of service from one community to another so the families and friends can continue to receive support after the PWA has died.

• Parish ministers, in particular, should work with hospitals, nursing homes, community agencies, and pastoral care services to assist them in dealing with PWAs and with their own feelings as they fulfill their ministerial duties. The spiritual care of PWAs and their loved ones is a call for us to respond in a special way throughout every level of Church ministry.

THE GOSPEL ALIVE

The Church has many resources—physical, financial, and spiritual—but its most important resource is people. The answer to AIDS will depend on people answering the call for assistance.

We have a responsibility to ensure that persons affected by AIDS are cared for compassionately with love and mercy. We have a responsibility to become facilitators, advocates, and conveners to make sure that unmet needs are addressed through collaboration and networking. We have a responsibility to be credible and to make our own policies, practices, and attitudes reflect the Gospel. We have a responsibility to make our institutions, our parishes, and our actions show justice and fairness, love, and compassion. We have a responsibility not to be judgmental, accusatory, or discriminating.

AIDS presents a unique set of psychological, social, moral, and spiritual issues. The Church will come alive as it awakens society to Jesus' love in this contemporary experience of AIDS. Our special concern for the poor, the marginated, the disenfranchised, and the sick can be demonstrated fully and clearly as we heed and are empowered by the Gospel's call to resolve the AIDS crisis. We are being called and empowered to teach and to heal. We are called and empowered to draw on our rich theological and moral tradition in shaping a Christian response to AIDS. We are called and empowered to serve one another and to help all persons achieve the potential that God has willed for them and ultimately for society as a whole.

Predictions of the effect of AIDS into the 1990s are absolutely staggering, particularly with regard to the number of affected women and children. Our call as a Catholic healthcare ministry is to demonstrate that the Gospel is alive in meeting the AIDS crisis:

> Ours is a ministry of bringing life, of healing brokenness, of confronting death—one in which people care for one another, comfort and touch one another, and often journey with one another into the very mystery of God's love—the hope of resurrection. This ministry is a concrete manifestation of the power of the risen Christ, here and now.[5]

NOTES

1. AIDS Project Los Angeles, "Biblical Perspective on AIDS," *AIDS: A Self Care Manual,* ed. Betty Clare Moffat, Judith Spiegel, Steve Parrish, and Michael Helquist, IBS Press, Santa Monica, CA, 1987, p. 224.
2. "Biblical Perspective on AIDS."
3. "Biblical Perspective on AIDS."
4. From CHA testimony on *The Many Faces of AIDS: A Gospel Response,* before the Episcopal Task Force of the National Conference of Catholic Bishops, Washington, DC, July 1987. See also United States Catholic Conference Administrative Board, "The Many Faces of AIDS: A Gospel Response," *Origins,* Dec. 24, 1987, pp. 4.
5. Sr. Mary Eileen Wilhelm speech to Pope John Paul II and The Catholic Health Association of the United States, Phoenix, AZ, Sept. 14, 1987.

Appendix

The following exhibits contain sample policies and procedures relating to various aspects of AIDS in the healthcare setting. These samples are not intended as "models," however. They are not offered as examples of how an organization's policy should look. They are not to be adopted blindly without discussion and the good counsel of qualified ethical, medical, nursing, and legal professionals. They are, simply, examples of the kinds of policies that some institutions have adopted. None is perfect; all can be improved. They should be read, discussed, dissected, adapted, or rejected according to the needs of the organization and its personnel. The sample policies are offered to encourage readers to prepare for AIDS-related problems before they arise. If that is done, the quality of care for persons with AIDS will be greatly enhanced.

SAMPLE POLICIES

Request for and Consent to AIDS Antibody Testing #1
Request for and Consent to AIDS Antibody Testing #2
Request for and Consent to AIDS Antibody Testing #3
Policies for Protection of All Healthcare Workers from
    Blood-Borne Infections
Employees with Acquired Immune Deficiency Syndrome (AIDS)
Employment and Patient Care Issues Related to AIDS
Infection Control Procedures
Corporate Policies
    Levi Strauss & Co.
    Pacific Gas and Electric Company
    Wells Fargo Bank
    San Francisco Chamber of Commerce

REQUEST FOR AND CONSENT TO AIDS ANTIBODY TESTING #1

I, _____, request and consent to undergo a blood test to detect whether I have antibodies in my blood to the acquired immune deficiency syndrome ("AIDS") virus. I have been informed that the test, which is performed by the drawing of blood sample, is currently the only method to detect exposure to AIDS and will be performed by _____ ("Laboratory"). If the test results are positive, Doctor will use other methods to determine whether I have AIDS.

Dr. _____ ("Doctor") has explained to me and I understand that a positive test result:

1. Is found in almost all persons with AIDS

2. May indicate that I have been infected by the AIDS virus and will be considered infectious (able to transmit the virus to other persons)

3. Does not necessarily mean that I have AIDS or will develop AIDS (many well people with a positive antibody test have not developed AIDS or AIDS related diseases; some have)

4. Will require that I consult with Doctor concerning the meaning of the test result and necessary future studies and/or tests

5. May require further testing and/or additional blood samples to confirm the results of the test

I further understand that AIDS antibody testing is not one hundred percent (100%) accurate and may, in some circumstances, indicate that a person has antibodies to the virus when the person does not (this is known as a false-positive), or fail to detect that a person has antibodies to the virus when the person, in fact, does have antibodies (this is known as a false-negative). If the result of the first test (ELISA) is positive, the Laboratory will perform a second test (Western Blot) to reduce the chances of a false positive.

Doctor has informed me, and I understand, that there is a lag time between the time that a person is exposed to the AIDS virus and the time that the AIDS antibodies first appear in the blood. As a result, I

Reprinted with the permission of SSM Health Care System.

understand that a negative test result does not necessarily mean that I have not been exposed to, or infected by, the AIDS virus.

I understand that my test results will become part of my medical record and, as such, will be accessible to physicians and other healthcare providers directly involved in my medical care, and may be disclosed as required by state and federal laws and regulations.

I request and give permission to have a blood sample taken for AIDS antibody testing. In consideration of the performance of this blood test and other consideration I have received, I hereby remise, release and discharge _____ which owns and operates _____, its medical staff, officers, directors, agents and employees and Doctor from any and all claims, demands, actions, and liability for any injury or damages which arise directly or indirectly from the necessary disclosure of the results thereof.

I have been informed concerning the risks and benefits relating to the AIDS antibody blood test as well as the alternatives to this test. By placing my signature below, I specifically acknowledge that I have been given all of the information that I need in order to make an informed decision regarding whether to undergo AIDS antibody testing, that I have had an opportunity to ask questions and that all of my questions have been answered.

_____

Patient, Parent, or Legal Guardian's Signature

a.m.
_____p.m.
Date   /   Time

REQUEST FOR AND CONSENT TO AIDS ANTIBODY TESTING #2

I, _____, request and consent to Dr. _____ ("Doctor") ordering a blood test to detect antibodies to the acquired immune deficiency syndrome ("AIDS") in my blood. I consent to the drawing of blood by Doctor or agents or employees of Healthcare Facility and to the testing of my blood by _____ ("Laboratory"). If the test results are positive, Doctor will use other methods to determine whether I have AIDS.

Dr. _____ ("Doctor") has explained to me and I understand that a positive test result:

1. Is found in almost all persons with AIDS

2. May indicate that I have been infected by the AIDS virus and will be considered infectious (able to transmit the virus to other persons)

3. Does not necessarily mean that I have AIDS or will develop AIDS (many well people with a positive antibody test have not developed AIDS or AIDS related diseases; some have)

4. Will require that I consult with Doctor concerning the meaning of the test result and necessary future studies and/or tests

5. May require further testing and/or additional blood samples to confirm the results of the test

I further understand that AIDS antibody testing is not one hundred percent (100%) accurate and may, in some circumstances, indicate that a person has antibodies to the virus when the person does not (this is known as a false-positive), or fail to detect that a person has antibodies to the virus when the person, in fact, does have antibodies (this is known as a false-negative). If the result of the first test (ELISA) is positive, the Laboratory will perform a second test (Western Blot) to reduce the chances of a false positive.

Doctor has informed me, and I understand, that there is a lag time between the time that a person is exposed to the AIDS virus and the time that the AIDS antibodies first appear in the blood. As a result, I understand that a negative test result does not necessarily mean that I have not been exposed to, or infected by, the AIDS virus.

I understand that my test results will become part of my medical record and, as such, will be accessible to physicians and other healthcare providers directly involved in my medical care, and may be disclosed as required by state and federal laws and regulations.

I request and give permission to have a blood sample taken for AIDS antibody testing. In consideration of the performance of this blood test and other consideration I have received, I hereby remise, release, and discharge _____ which owns and operates _____, its medical staff, officers, directors, agents and employees and Doctor from any and all claims, demands, actions, and liability for any injury or damages which arise directly or indirectly from the necessary disclosure of the results thereof.

I have been informed concerning the risks and benefits relating to the AIDS antibody blood test as well as the alternatives to this test. By placing my signature below, I specifically acknowledge that I have been given all of the information that I need in order to make an informed decision regarding whether to undergo AIDS antibody testing, that I have had an opportunity to ask questions and that all of my questions have been answered.

_____

Patient, Parent, or Legal Guardian's Signature

                                                        a.m.
_____ p.m.
          Date   /   Time

_____

Witness

_____

Physician Acknowledgment

I, _____, hereby acknowledge that I
have explained to the above-named patient the nature of the ELISA
and Western Blot Tests, their necessity, expected benefits, risks and
alternatives.

_____
Physician's Signature

                                                        a.m.
_____p.m.
        Date   /   Time

REQUEST FOR AND CONSENT TO AIDS ANTIBODY TESTING #3

I, _____, request and consent to Dr. _____ ("Doctor") ordering a blood test to detect antibodies to the acquired immune deficiency syndrome ("AIDS") in my blood. I consent to the drawing of blood by Doctor or agents or employees of Healthcare Facility and to the testing of my blood by _____ ("Laboratory").

Doctor has explained to me, and I understand, that this test will show whether I have been exposed to AIDS but will not show whether I have or will get AIDS. There are currently no other means to detect exposure to AIDS. If the test result is positive, Doctor will use other means to determine whether I have AIDS.

Doctor has informed me that the tests for the AIDS antibody are new and their accuracy and reliability are still uncertain. The results may, in rare cases, indicate that a person has antibodies to AIDS when the person does not (false positive) or fail to detect that a person has antibodies to AIDS when the person has antibodies (false negative). If the result of the first test (ELISA) is positive, the Laboratory will perform a second test (Western Blot), to reduce the chances of a false positive.

Doctor has informed me, and I understand, that there is a lag time between the time that a person is exposed to the AIDS virus and the time that the AIDS antibodies first appear in the blood. As a result, I understand that a negative test result does not necessarily mean that I have not been exposed to, or infected by, the AIDS virus.

I understand that my test results will become part of my medical records and, as such, will be accessible to physicians and other healthcare providers directly involved in my medical care, and may be disclosed as required by state and federal laws and regulations.

Doctor has explained to me, and I understand, that the blood test is necessary because _____ _____. The withdrawal of blood may cause slight bruising, swelling or a local infection in the area where the needle pierces the skin.

Reprinted with the permission of SSM Health Care System.

I have had an opportunity to read this form and Doctor has answered all of my questions satisfactorily regarding the nature of the blood test, its expected benefits, risks, and alternatives.

_____
Patient, Parent, or Legal Guardian's Signature

                                                     a.m.
_____p.m.
        Date   /   Time

_____
Witness

_____
Physician Acknowledgment

I, _____, hereby acknowledge that I have explained to the above-named patient the nature of the ELISA and Western Blot Tests, their necessity, expected benefits, risks, and alternatives.

_____
Physician's Signature

                                                     a.m.
_____p.m.
        Date   /   Time

POLICIES FOR PROTECTION OF ALL HEALTHCARE WORKERS FROM BLOOD-BORNE INFECTIONS

In keeping with recommendations from both the Centers for Disease Control and the American Hospital Association, for the purposes of protecting, insofar as possible, all healthcare workers at Healthcare Facility from infectious diseases transmitted by blood and body fluids, the following policies shall apply to all persons at Healthcare Facility:

A. *All Personnel.*

    1. *Blood and Bodily Fluid Precautions.* Strict adherence to all standard infection control policies pertaining to obtaining and handling of patient specimens shall be maintained. Appropriate isolation will be ordered and observed whenever specific infectious diseases are suspected or diagnosed. Patients for whom isolation is ordered, their equipment, and all specimens from such patients will be so labelled.

    2. *Universal Precautions.* Blood and body fluids from *all patients,* whether previously identified and isolated or not, shall be considered potentially infectious and appropriate precautions taken by personnel handling or anticipating exposure to these specimens. These universal precautions are particularly important for persons in the Emergency Department.

        (a) *Barrier Precautions.* Equipment for barrier protection shall be conveniently available in areas of patient care.

            (i) *Gloves.* Gloves should be worn for touching blood and body fluids, mucous membranes, or non-intact skin of all patients, for handling items or surfaces soiled with blood or body fluids, and for performing venipuncture and other vascular access procedures. Gloves must be changed between each patient contact.

            (ii) *Masks.* Masks and protective eyewear or face shields should be worn during procedures likely to generate droplets of blood or other body fluids.

            (iii) *Gowns.* Gowns should be worn during procedures

likely to generate splashes of blood or other body fluids.

(b) *Hand Washing.* Hands and other skin surfaces should be washed immediately and thoroughly if contaminated with blood or other body fluids. Hands should be washed immediately after gloves and gowns are removed.

(c) *Prevent Injuries.* All persons should take precautions to prevent injuries caused by needles, scalpels, and other sharp instruments. Needles should not be recapped, purposely bent or broken by hand, removed from disposable syringes, or otherwise manipulated by hand. After use, disposable syringes and needles, scalpel blades, and other sharp items should be placed in puncture-resistant containers for disposal. Large-bore reusable needles should be placed in a puncture-resistant container for transport to the reprocessing area. Only needle-locking syringes or one-piece needle-syringe units should be used to aspirate fluids from patients, so that collected fluid can be safely discharged through the needle, if desired.

(d) *Blood Spills.* Blood spills should be cleaned up promptly with a disinfectant solution.

(e) *Resuscitation Precautions.* To minimize mouth-to-mouth resuscitation, persons should use mouthpieces, resuscitation bags, or other ventilation devices.

(f) *Unsafe Patient Contact.* Persons with exudative lesions or weeping dermatitis should refrain from all direct patient care and from handling patient-care equipment until the condition resolves.

B. *Precautions for Invasive Procedures.*

1. *Definition of "Invasive Procedure."* For purposes of these policies, invasive procedure is defined as surgical entry into tissues, cavities, or organs or repair of major traumatic injuries (a) in an operating room, the Emergency Department, or the Outpatient Department; (b) cardiac catheterization and angiographic procedures; (c) the manipulation, cutting, or removal of any oral or perioral tissues, including tooth structure, during which bleeding occurs or the potential for bleeding exists.

   Persons involved in invasive procedures should adhere to the universal precautions set forth earlier in this policy in addition to the precautions set forth below:

2. *Gloves and Masks.* Gloves and surgical masks *must* be worn for all invasive procedures.

3. *Protective Eyewear.* Protective eyewear or face shields should be worn for procedures that commonly result in the generation of droplets, splashing of blood or other body fluids, or the generation of bone chips.

4. *Gowns or Aprons.* Gowns or aprons made of materials that provide an effective barrier should be worn during invasive procedures that are likely to result in the splashing of blood or other body fluids.

5. *Injuries.* If a glove is torn or a needlestick or other surgery occurs, replace the glove as promptly as patient safety permits. Remove the needle or instrument involved from the sterile field.

C. *Precautions for Autopsies.* Persons performing postmortem procedures should adhere to the universal precautions set forth earlier in these policies in addition to the precautions set forth below:

1. *Barrier Protection.* All persons performing or assisting in postmortem procedures should wear gloves, masks, protective eyewear, gowns and waterproof aprons, and waterproof shoe coverings.

2. *Contaminated Materials.* Instruments and surfaces contaminated during postmortem procedures should be decontaminated with an appropriate chemical germicide.

D. *Precautions for Laboratories.* Persons working in the labs should adhere to the universal precautions set forth earlier in these policies in addition to the precautions set forth below:

1. *Containers.* All specimens of blood and body fluids should be put in a well-constructed container with a secure lid to prevent leaking during transport. Care should be taken when collecting each specimen to avoid contaminating the outside of the container and of the laboratory form accompanying the specimen.

2. *Gloves and Masks.* All persons processing blood and body-fluid specimens (e.g., removing tops from vacuum tubes) should

wear gloves. Masks and protective eyewear should be worn if mucous-membrane contact with blood or body fluids is anticipated. Gloves should be changed and hands washed after completion of specimen processing.

3. *Biological Safety Cabinets.* For routine procedures, such as histologic and pathologic studies or microbiologic culturing, a biological safety cabinet is not necessary. However, biological safety cabinets (Class I or II) should be used whenever procedures are conducted that have a high potential for generating droplets. These include activities such as blending, sonicating, and vigorous mixing.

4. *Mechanical Pipetting Devices.* Mechanical pipetting devices should be used for manipulating all liquids in the laboratory. Mouth pipetting must not be done.

5. *Needles and Syringes.* Use of needles and syringes should be limited to situations in which there is no alternative, and the recommendations for preventing injuries with needles outlined under the universal precautions should be followed.

6. *Blood Spills.* Laboratory work surfaces should be decontaminated with an appropriate chemical germicide after a spill of blood or other body fluids and when work activities are completed.

7. *Contaminated Materials.* Contaminated materials used in laboratory tests should be decontaminated before reprocessing or be placed in bags and disposed of in accordance with Healthcare Facility's policies for disposal of infective waste. Scientific equipment that has been contaminated with blood or other body fluids should be decontaminated and cleaned before being repaired in the laboratory or transported to the manufacturer.

8. *Hand Washing.* All persons should wash their hands after completing laboratory activities and should remove protective clothing before leaving the laboratory.

E. *Housekeeping.*

1. *Blood Spills.* Blood spills should be cleaned up promptly with a disinfectant solution, such as sodium hypochlorite.

2. *Linens.* Articles soiled with blood should be placed in an impervious bag prominently labeled "Blood Precautions" before

being sent for reprocessing or disposal. Alternatively, such contaminated items may be placed in plastic bags of a particular color designated solely for disposal of infectious wastes. Reusable items should be reprocessed pursuant to Healthcare Facility's policies for hepatitis B virus-contaminated items.

3. *Gloves.* Gloves should always be worn during cleaning and decontaminating procedures.

F. *Management of Exposures.* Any person who has a parenteral (e.g., needlestick or cut) or mucous-membrane (e.g., splash to the eye or mouth) exposure to blood or other body fluids or has a cutaneous exposure involving large amounts of blood or prolonged contact with blood, especially when the exposed skin is chapped, abraded, or afflicted with dermatitis, should notify his or her department director who shall counsel the exposed person on risk of infection and arrange appropriate testing for infection, if the exposed person consents. The department director shall document the exposure, that counselling was given and the serologic testing performed, if any.

G. *Reporting Requirements.*

1. *Reports to the Department of Health.*

    (a) *Attending Physician.* The attending physician of a patient who has or is suspected of having AIDS, Hepatitis A, B and non-A, non-B or who is HIV seropositive shall report the following information to the Department of Health within seven (7) days of the suspected or established diagnosis: (i) name; (ii) address; (iii) age; (iv) sex; (v) race; (vi) name of the disease or condition diagnosed or suspected and the date of onset of the illness.

    (b) *Healthcare Facility.* The attending physician may authorize, in writing, the executive director or his or her designee to make the report required in Section 1(a) regarding a patient who is currently an inpatient at Healthcare Facility. Such report must include, in addition to the information set forth in 1(a), (i) the name and address of the hospital; (ii) the date of the report; (iii) the name and address of the attending physician; (iv) and any appropriate laboratory results.

(c) *Laboratories.* Laboratories processing tests for HIV sero-positivity or hepatitis must submit the following information to the Department of Health within seven (7) days: (i) the test performed; (ii) the test results; (iii) the name and address of the attending physician; (iv) the name of the disease or condition diagnosed or suspected; (v) the date the test results were obtained; and (vi) the patient's name, sex, age, and race.

2. *Notice to Patient, Family, and Attendants.* The attending physician immediately upon diagnosing a case of a reportable communicable disease, must give detailed instructions to the patient, members of the household, and attendants regarding proper control measures.

3. *Death of a Person with a Communicable Disease.* When a person dies while infected with a communicable disease, the attending physician shall notify the funeral director, embalmer, or other responsible person regarding the communicable disease the deceased had at the time of death. A tag shall be affixed to the body indicating the name of the communicable disease likely to have been present at the time of death.

H. *Education.* Information, education, and in-service training on the epidemiology, modes of transmission, and prevention of HIV and other blood-borne infections and the need for routine use of universal blood and body-fluid precautions for *all* patients shall be incorporated into the educational programs of all personnel, including the medical staff.

I. *Corrective Action.* The failure of any person to adhere to these policies may result in corrective or disciplinary action.

Formulated: _____

EMPLOYEES WITH ACQUIRED IMMUNE DEFICIENCY SYNDROME (AIDS)

A. *Policy.* In making employment decisions which affect an existing or prospective employee diagnosed as having acquired immune deficiency syndrome ("AIDS"), AIDS related complex ("ARC"), human immunodeficiency virus ("HIV") seropositivity, or some secondary infection, Healthcare Facility must consider its legal obligations not to discriminate against handicapped persons in conjunction with the responsibility to provide quality healthcare services to patients and to exercise reasonable care to provide a safe working environment for all employees. Healthcare Facility shall make employment decisions regarding persons with AIDS, ARC, HIV seropositivity, or some secondary infection on an individual basis. Such decisions shall be based on:

1. The person's ability to perform his or her duties

2. Healthcare Facility's ability to make reasonable accommodations to the person's medical condition, including necessary precautions to minimize risks posed by the person's condition

3. The harm the duties of the job may present to the person

4. Considering the duties of the job, the recognized medical harm the person may present to others, including co-workers and patients

5. Any relevant laws or regulations

In consideration of these obligations, Healthcare Facility has adopted this policy and the following guidelines to deal with an employee or applicant for employment who has or may have AIDS, ARC, or HIV seropositivity. This policy has been prepared pursuant to the current status of the law in this area and medical knowledge regarding the disease and may be affected by future developments in the law or medicine.

(a) Healthcare Facilty shall apply existing personnel policies and procedures regarding employment, working conditions, dismissal, sick leave, termination of employment and

Reprinted with the permission of SSM Health Care System.

related matters to employees diagnosed with AIDS, ARC, HIV seropositivity, or some secondary infection (i) on the same basis as to employees who have other diseases or conditions which may incapacitate them for work or otherwise affect job performance and (ii) in a manner which is consistent with or required by local, state, and federal laws and regulations.

(b) Healthcare Facility shall provide insurance and other benefits to employees diagnosed with AIDS, ARC, HIV seropositivity, or some secondary infection in accordance with existing employee benefit plans, if such employees otherwise satisfy the eligibility and co-payment requirements, if any, applicable under existing or future employee benefit plans.

(c) Employees with AIDS, ARC, HIV seropositivity, or some secondary infection who have the ability to perform their jobs without putting others at risk of infection may work without restriction. If, however, such employees show signs of an infection or illness which could expose others to a medically recognized risk of infection, then Healthcare Facility shall require them to take a mandatory medical leave of absence. Such employees shall not return to work until such time as Healthcare Facility has medical evidence to its satisfaction that they no longer could expose others to a medically recognized risk of infection.

(d) Employees who refuse to work with co-workers or patients with a diagnosis of AIDS, ARC, HIV seropositivity, or a secondary infection without approved exemption, as provided below in paragraph (e), may subject themselves to corrective action, which may include the termination of employment.

(e) Healthcare Facility may excuse pregnant or immunosuppressed employees who are more susceptible to certain viruses (i.e., cytomegalovirus) from working with persons with AIDS. Employees who desire to be excused from working with persons with AIDS pursuant to this paragraph should present medical documentation and a recommendation from a physician selected by or acceptable to

Healthcare Facility that such exemption is medically necessary.

(f) Healthcare Facility shall not routinely require serologic blood testing of employment applicants or current employees. If a situation arises in which Healthcare Facility considers a blood test to be appropriate, such testing shall not occur without the employee's prior written consent. However, if an employee refuses either to submit to a blood test or to release the test's results to Healthcare Facility, or both, when requested by Healthcare Facility, the hospital may take corrective action against the employee, which may include the termination of employment.

(g) Healthcare Facility shall refrain from taking into account an individual's association with a person with AIDS in any decisions to hire, to promote, to transfer, to evaluate job performance, to adjust wages, to assign work, to change working conditions, or to dismiss.

(h) Healthcare Facility shall not terminate the employment of an employee with AIDS or a related condition because of or to prevent a claim against such employee's retirement benefits.

(i) Any supervisor, medical staff member or other person who receives information regarding an employee's diagnosis of AIDS, ARC, HIV seropositivity, or a secondary infection shall only disclose such information to those who need to know to fulfill his or her job or legal responsibilities.

(j) An employee physician who diagnoses AIDS pursuant to the current CDC definition of AIDS is required by law to and will report such diagnosis to the state department of health.

(k) Healthcare Facility will make employee assistance program ("EAP") services available to employees with AIDS, ARC or HIV seropositivity.

B. *Procedure.*

1. The department director should discuss the employee's current health status in confidence with that individual.

   (a) Review the employee's assessment as to his or her ability and desire to work.

(b) Reassure the employee that Healthcare Facility will attempt to work in conjunction with the employee and his or her personal physician to accommodate the disability to the extent that is possible.

(c) Ensure that the employee is aware of Healthcare Facility's leave of absence policy should long term absences become necessary.

2. Request that the employee sign a "Consent to Release of Medical Records" to be given to the individual's treating physician and/or any other physician or healthcare facility which might maintain the applicable medical records regarding the individual's current condition.

(a) Advise the employee that the purpose of contacting the employee's treating physician is to enable a dialogue between Healthcare Facility and the physician to determine whether the employee is physically able to perform the full range of his or her job duties and that the employee's continued performance in his or her current position is medically appropriate.

(b) Ensure that the employee understands that this information will be kept confidential and released only to persons acting on behalf of Healthcare Facility on a "need to know" basis.

3. In conjunction with the employee, discuss and evaluate the employee's ability to perform job duties adequately and safely.

(a) Assess limitations, including hazards which impact on the employee's own health due to the potential for exposure to infection, as well as in terms of the safe delivery of patient care (e.g., responsibility for participation in invasive procedures).

(b) Consider possibilities available for alternate assignments, if appropriate.

(c) After reviewing concerns and options with the employee, propose arrangements which will best serve the needs of all concerned.

4. Send a copy of the employee's job description, revised as necessary and a signed "Consent to Release of Medical Records" to the employee's treating physician. Request that the

physician review the duties in terms of the patient's physical condition and advise Healthcare Facility in writing of the following:

(a) Whether it is medically appropriate for the employee to return to work within the hospital environment.

(b) Whether he or she is able to perform the full range of job responsibilities; and if not, to specify what limitations are recommended.

(c) Whether any protective measures — aside from normal precautionary measures prescribed by hospital policy — should be utilized.

(d) Confirmation that the employee's performance of the duties described within a hospital environment will not pose undue risk to patients or co-workers, providing recommended precautionary measures are followed.

(e) An agreement that the physician will contact Healthcare Facility if the employee's condition changes, including the development of a secondary infection.

5. If deemed appropriate by Healthcare Facility, review the circumstances of the employee's return to or continuation of work — including the statement from the employee's physician and the intended job description — with a qualified medical professional acting on behalf of Healthcare Facility. Obtain a written statement from such physician which confirms that it is medically appropriate for the employee to perform the duties outlined within the limitations specified; that working within the hospital environment does not pose undue risk to the employee; and that the employee's return to work will not pose undue risk to patients or other employees at Healthcare Facility.

If the opinions of the employee's treating physician and the physician acting on behalf of Healthcare Facility are not consistent, Healthcare Facility may obtain the opinion of an independent physician agreed upon by Healthcare Facility and the employee's treating physician.

6. Review the medical recommendations secured with the employee. Ensure that he or she understands that continuing to work in the hospital environment increases the chance of

contracting an infection which, because of the condition of his or her health, could be life threatening. If necessary, provide counselling for the employee with regard to precautionary measures, such as CDC recommendations to minimize the risk of infection to the employee involving exposure to patients with infectious diseases; and guidelines to prevent transmission from the employee to patients.

7. Require that the employee sign a statement which releases Healthcare Facility from liability which may be incurred as a result of the employee's decision to continue his or her employment. This statement should also confirm that the employee agrees to keep Healthcare Facility apprised of any changes in his or her physical condition which may impact on his or her ability to perform any and all required duties or which may pose a risk to the health of others (e.g., the development of a secondary infection).

EMPLOYMENT AND PATIENT CARE ISSUES RELATED TO AIDS

Acquired immune deficiency syndrome (AIDS) has become a major health issue for healthcare professionals and the general public since it was first reported in 1981. Further, the incidence of AIDS is increasing and the disease will likely remain a significant health problem into the foreseeable future. The following address certain employment and patient care issues related to AIDS.

A. *Policy*

All operating entities (*) will:

1. treat patients with AIDS or AIDS-related complex (ARC) with the same compassion, competence, and understanding as other patients

2. follow ethical principles for terminally ill AIDS patients in the final stages of their illness

3. attend to the social, psychological, spiritual, emotional, as well as, physical needs of AIDS patients coping with imminent death, the news of an AIDS diagnosis or exposure to the HIV virus, and the choices that such patients must make

4. maintain confidentiality (to include special handling of medical records, if appropriate) of all patients with AIDS, ARC, or seropositivity for the antibody to AIDS

5. comply with applicable federal, state, and municipal laws, regulations and reporting requirements in the treatment of patients, employees, and prospective employees with AIDS

(*) The employment aspects of this policy are applicable to all operating entities. Naturally, the patient care aspects of the policy are applicable to those operating entities engaged in patient care services.

Reprinted with the permission of the SSM Health Care System.

6. maintain a safe working place and patient care environment in accordance with guidelines from the Centers for Disease Control (CDC) and/or other professional/clinical organizations and applicable federal, state, and local laws and regulations

7. insure that all appropriate precautions are taken as they relate to autopsies, blood and blood products, and donation/ transplantation of tissues, organs, and body fluids

B. *Attachment*

The attachment to this policy provides additional information and guidelines on the AIDS issue relating to patient care and employment.

ADDITIONAL INFORMATION AND GUIDELINES ON AIDS

The following additional information and guidelines are reflective of present knowledge about AIDS. It is subject to change as more information becomes available.

Patient Care Issues

1. The medical staff or operating entity, through its established mechanisms, should determine the indications and criteria for ordering laboratory screening tests for AIDS and seropositivity to the HIV virus and blood and body fluid precautions. More definitive tests (i.e., Western Blot) should be used to confirm seropositive patients.

2. The patient's written informed consent will be obtained before AIDS and HIV virus screening tests are conducted. Informal consent will be obtained by the physician. Such written consent should become part of the patient's medical record.

3. AIDS or ARC diagnosis or seropositivity should be documented in the patient's medical record by the physician.

4. Placement of an AIDS patient in a private room, though not necessarily required, may be indicated to protect the patient from infections or to protect the patient's confidentiality.

5. Pulmonary resuscitation equipment (ambu bag and oral airway) will be immediately available for use on patients with AIDS, ARC, or HIV seropositivity.

6. Information regarding seropositive test results or a diagnosis of AIDS or ARC should only be disclosed as necessary for patient care, employer protection, and federal, state, and local reporting requirements.

7. AIDS, ARC and HIV seropositive patients will receive appropriate counseling and education to prevent spreading the HIV virus.

Employment Issues

1. Employees are expected to carry out their duties toward the care of all patients. Employees who refuse to treat patients with AIDS,

ARC, or HIV positivity, without approved exemption, may subject themselves to appropriate disciplinary action.

2. All employees are expected to provide care or job-related activities for patients who are isolated for a communicable disease or infectious condition. As long as proper precautions are observed, employees are not at risk. All employees must be aware that all patients are potentially infectious and care should be taken to avoid transmission of disease. Policies and procedures regarding infectious diseases and exemption of employees caring for patients with infectious diseases will be dealt with on an individual case-by-case basis at the employing facility.

3. Employees and applicants for employment should not be routinely tested for the AIDS antibody in pre-employment and periodic employment physicals and, in any case, never without a prior written informed consent.

4. Procedures for dealing with injuries to an employee (such as needle sticks), which may expose the employee to the HIV virus should include:

   a. Available testing for the employee for the HIV antibody at periodic intervals to be determined by the employee health physician or a physician designated by the operating entity

   b. Informing the employee of the results of any tests in appropriate and timely manner

   c. Maintaining all information in confidence except to the extent disclosure is required by law or is necessary for determination of the employee's duties in the work place

   d. Counseling and advisory services as appropriate to the employee's situation

NOTE: These situations should be dealt with on a case-by-case basis. Insurance and compensation benefits for these employees are provided in accordance with existing employee compensation guidelines.

Other Considerations

1. Social services in each operating entity should be aware of all AIDS treatment programs in the community to assist patients with AIDS in referral to appropriate treatment resources (long term care, home case, hospice, etc.).

2. Operating entities should work with public health agencies and health education groups to provide accurate and timely information about AIDS to the community and to employees. Awareness programs should include:

   a. possible medical procedures that are available

   b. appropriate referral to facilities where care may be available

   c. appropriate counseling and support services necessary to help people deal with the knowledge of AIDS and to make appropriate and intelligent decisions

3. The social and ethical implications of AIDS should be considered in all educational materials and presentations. Resources are available in the corporate services office to assist operating entities in developing educational programs on AIDS.

INFECTION CONTROL PROCEDURES

A. *Patient Care Practices*

The following are the precautions necessary for the care of a patient with acquired immune deficiency syndrome (AIDS). For the patient with additional infectious complications, it may also be necessary to institute other precautions. To determine if additional precautions are necessary, medical and nursing personnel should consult the Centers for Disease Control (CDC) Guidelines for Isolation Precautions in Hospitals, which can be found in Section H of the Nursing Policy and Procedure Manual.

1. *Handwashing*

   a. *Handwashing is the single most important means of preventing the spread of infection.*

   b. Hands must be washed before and after all patient contact, as well as after eating and using the lavatory.

   c. Strict handwashing must also be practiced immediately after becoming contaminated with blood, and after removal of gown and gloves.

2. *Gloves*

   a. Gloves must be worn for all contact with blood, blood soiled items, body fluids, excretions and secretions, or contaminated articles.

3. *Masks*

   a. Masks are not routinely necessary for the care of patients with AIDS.

   b. The use of masks is recommended in the following situations:

   • When healthcare workers (HCWs) have direct, sustained contact with a patient who is coughing extensively or a patient who is intubated or being suctioned

   • To protect the patient when the HCW has a cold or other active upper respiratory tract infection

   • When the patient has tuberculosis (TB). When TB is

Reprinted with permission of St. Clare Hospital, New York.

suspected or confirmed, masks must be worn until there are 3 consecutive sputum smears which are negative for AFB (acid-fast bacilli). This usually occurs within 2-3 weeks after chemotherapy is begun.

4. *Gowns*

   a. Gowns must be worn when clothes may become soiled, or when having *direct contact* with patients' blood soiled items, body fluids, excretions and secretions, or with contaminated articles.

5. *Private Room*

   a. A private room is necessary for a patient with poor hygiene (i.e., when the patient does not wash hands after touching infective material, contaminates the environment with infective material, or shares contaminated articles with other patients).

   b. A patient with AIDS may share a room with another patient with AIDS, as long as they are matched according to their opportunistic infections. Similarly, these complications are considered not to be transmissible to others, and thus patients with such may be placed in two-bed rooms:

   • Kaposi's sarcoma (KS) and other AIDS associated neoplasma
   • Candidiasis esophagitis
   • Cryptococcal miningitis
   • Mycobacterium avium intracellulare (MAI)
   • Cytomegalovirus (CMV) retinitis
   • Central nervous system (CNS) toxoplasmosis

   c. A patient with AIDS may also share a room with a non-AIDS patient, as long as that non-AIDS patient is not immunosuppressed or infected with potentially transmissible pathogens.

   d. A private room may also be necessary if indicated by the patient's physician.

6. *Transporting Patients*

   a. Patients being transported to other areas of the hospital require no special precautions, other than those routinely applied when the HCW enters the patient's room. However, when the patient is being transported, the patient, rather than the HCW, takes the necessary precautions.

   b. Generally, the only precaution necessary is the use of masks for the patient with tuberculosis, in order to prevent the airborne spread of acid-fast bacilli. (Masks become less efficient as they become moistened, and thus should be changed after approximately 20 minutes. Personnel should therefore carry additional masks with them when transporting such patients, and must dispose of used masks as infectious waste.)

   c. Personnel in the area to which the patient is being transported should be informed that they must apply precautions for contact with blood and body fluids.

B. *Visitors*

  1. Visitors must follow the guidelines for isolation precautions which are outlined in items 1-4 under the heading of "Patient Care Practices."

  2. It is the responsibility of the nurse to explain the indicated precautions, and to instruct visitors on the use of gloves, masks, and gowns where appropriate.

C. *Care and Use of Equipment*

  1. *Needles and Syringes*

    a. Always use caution when handling needles and syringes, in order to avoid accidental needlesticks.

    b. Puncture-proof needle disposal containers are placed in all patient rooms, as well as other areas (e.g., treatment room, medication room) where needles may be used.

    c. Used needles must *never* be bent, clipped, or recapped after use; they should, instead, be placed in puncture-proof needle disposal containers immediately after use.

  2. *Sphygmomanometer and Stethescope*

    a. No special precautions are necessary unless contaminated by blood or other body fluids.

    b. Articles which become visibly contaminated should be wiped clean with a 1:10 dilution of sodium hypochlorite.

  3. *Thermometers*

    a. IVAC thermometers with disposable covers are used for taking patients' temperatures.

b. Disposable covers are disposed of inside the patient's room as infectious waste.

c. If IVAC apparatus becomes visibly contaminated with blood or body fluids, it should be wiped clean with a 1:10 dilution of sodium hypochlorite.

4. *Patient's Chart*

a. The chart should not be allowed to come in contact with infective material or objects which may be contaminated with infective material.

b. If chart becomes visibly contaminated with infective material, it should be wiped clean with a 1:10 dilution of sodium hypochlorite.

5. *Code Cart*

a. The code cart is stored in the treatment room and taken into the patient's room when a code is called.

b. After the code is completed, the code cart is reviewed to assure that all used materials have been properly disposed of.

c. The code cart and intubation equipment are then cleaned with a 1:10 dilution of sodium hypochlorite.

d. The entire code cart is then returned to Central Supply for replacement of supplies.

6. *Decontamination of Reusable Equipment*

a. In general, invasive patient care equipment should be disposable or should be sterilized. More specifically:

- Laryngoscopes, bronchoscopes, endoscopes, endotracheal tubes, and other instruments that come in contact with blood, secretions, excretions, or tissues should be sterilized before reuse.

- Lensed instruments should be sterilized by ethylene oxide.

- Ventilator tubing must be disposable or sterilized before reuse.

7. *Dishes*

a. No special precautions are necessary for dishes, unless visibly contaminated with infective material.

b. Reusable dishes, utensils, and trays contaminated with infective material should be bagged and labelled before being returned to the food service department. Dietary personnel handling these trays and dishes should wear gloves, and should wash their hands before handling clean dishes or food.

8. *Linen*

   a. Used linen must be double bagged. It should first be placed in a water soluble bag and then in a red bag. The outside of the red bag must remain free from contamination, and must be closed securely.

   b. Red linen bags may be deposited in the laundry chute on each floor.

D. *Laboratory Specimens*

   1. Containers with blood and other specimens are to be completely enclosed within a clean plastic bag for transport. Both the outside of the specimen container and bag should remain clean and must be marked "Isolation Precautions."

   2. All labels and requisition slips on specimens must be marked "Isolation Precautions."

   3. If the outside of the specimen container is visibly contaminated with blood, it should be cleaned with a 1:10 dilution of sodium hypochlorite (household bleach/chlorox).

E. *Disposal of Infectious Wastes*

   1. *Isolation Garb*

      a. Upon removal of isolation garb (i.e., gowns, gloves, masks), place all garb in waste container *inside* the patient's room.

      • Isolation garb must never be worn in the hallways.

      • The same isolation garb must never be worn for the care of more than one patient.

      b. Hands must be washed after the removal of the above.

   2. *Infectious Waste*

      a. Disposable needles and syringes, scalpel blades, and other sharp items must always be deposited in puncture-proof needle disposal containers.

      • Puncture-proof needle disposal containers must be closed when they are three-quarters full, in order to prevent accidental needlesticks.

- Closed containers are stored in soiled utility room, to be collected by housekeeping personnel.

b. All liquid wastes are discarded directly into the sewage system (i.e., sink, drains, toilet, etc.).

c. All other wastes (e.g., isolation garb, dressings) are discarded in red plastic bags. Red bags must be double-bagged in a second red bag, which is then tied securely and held in the soiled utility room, to be picked up by housekeeping personnel.

F. *Patient Rooms*

Daily Cleaning and Disinfecting

1. *Policy*

Housekeeping staff should follow the same precautionary guidelines as those for employees who do not come into direct patient contact. Therefore, gowns and masks are not routinely required for cleaning of the room. If additional measures are needed, such instructions are indicated on the patient's door (e.g., Respiratory precautions may require masks).

2. *Procedure*

a. Wear appropriate protective apparel according to procedures outlined in policy on use of protective apparel.

b. Nursing personnel should clean all utensils and change the linen, using proper bagging techniques.

c. No wall washing or airing of the room is needed. If the case is extremely long term or walls are grossly soiled, some interim wall washing may be necessary, but only for spot cleaning.

d. Housekeeper will perform all of the duties outlined for terminal cleaning except washing the bed, making the bed, and cleaning the interior of drawers.

e. Remove protective apparel according to procedures outlined in policy on use of protective apparel.

f. Spills of blood and other body secretions should be cleaned up promptly. Large spills should be cleaned up by a gloved employee, using paper towels which should then be placed in an infectious waste container. Then any disinfectant-detergent solution, such as a fresh 1:10 dilution of 5.25 percent sodium hypochlorite with water, should be used to disinfect the area.

Terminal Cleaning

1. *Policy*

There shall be special procedures for cleaning a room after each patient is discharged.

2. *Procedure*

    a. Nursing personnel should remove all personal effects, utensils, and linen. Utensils (such as bedpans and urinals) should be emptied, bagged in red-impervious plastic and sent to central service for decontamination unless they are disposable, in which case they should be disposed of as contaminated waste. Linen should be double-bagged. Disposables should be placed in red-plastic bags or waste container liners.

    b. Housekeeper should remove drapes and cubicle curtains when indicated, (consider parameters used for wall cleaning) and double-bag them as isolation linen. If necessary, walls should be washed using Wall Glide Pro and Glide Rine Disinfectant (2 ounces per gallon of water).

    c. Housekeeper will perform the terminal cleaning procedure using the standard facility fresh solution (1:10 dilution of 5.25 percent sodium hypochlorite with water), and clean mops and cloths. Generally, standard check-out room cleaning procedures will be followed.

- Empty waste containers and ash trays. Trash should be double-bagged. Wash container and reline with a red plastic liner.
- High dusting: standard procedure
- Floor dusting: standard procedure
- Bed disinfection: standard procedure
- Furniture disinfection: standard procedure. This includes the bedside table, overbed table, dresser, desk, chairs, window ledges, electrical cords, telephone, etc.
- Spot clean walls, door handles, and door frames
- Clean the washroom: standard procedure
- Make the bed
- Sanitize the floor: with SaniMaster II, SaniMaster phenolic or Duoclene.
- Replace and straighten furniture

G. *Laboratories*

Precautions in Clinical Laboratories

1. The precautions to be taken in clinical laboratories are essentially the same as those recommended for processing specimens from patients known to be carriers of HBSAg.

2. Mechanical pipetting devices must be used for the manipulation of all liquids in the laboratory. Mouth pipetting must not be allowed.

3. Needles and syringes should be handled as described previously.

4. Laboratory coats, gowns, or uniforms should be worn while working with potentially infectious materials and should be removed before leaving the laboratory.

5. Gloves should be worn when handling blood, tissue specimens, blood soiled items, body fluids, excretions, and secretions, as well as surfaces, materials, and objects contaminated by them.

6. All procedures and manipulations of potentially infectious material should be performed in order to minimize the creation of droplets and aerosols. Procedures that have a high potential for creating aerosols or infectious droplets include centrifuging, blending, sonicating, vigorous mixing, and harvesting infected tissues from animals or embyonated eggs. Such procedures should be carried out in biological safety cabinets (class II). Whenever centrifugation of blood or body fluids from AIDS patients if necessary, the use of centrifuge safety cups is recommended.

7. Eating, drinking, and smoking should be prohibited in the immediate laboratory area.

8. Laboratory work surfaces should be decontaminated with a disinfectant, such as sodium hypochlorite solution, prepared as outlined previously, on a daily basis and following any spill of potentially infectious material.

9. Infectious waste from the laboratory should be processed according to established hospital policy for disposal of infectious waste.

10. Tissue or serum specimens to be stored should be clearly and permanently labeled as potentially hazardous.

11. All personnel should wash their hands following completion of laboratory activities, after removal of protective clothing and before leaving the laboratory.

H. *Autopsies*

Autopsy Precautions

The following recommendations for AIDS autopsy precautions are adapted from the joint recommendations of the Centers for Disease Control and the College of American Pathologists:

> As part of immediate post-mortem care, patients with AIDS or suspect AIDS should be identified "infectious hazard (blood/body fluid precautions)" and that identification should remain with the body whether or not an autopsy is carried out, for delivery to morticians.

> Double gloves, protective eye covering, masks, cap and gown and a waterproof apron and show coverings should be worn by personnel performing or viewing an autopsy in order to prevent parenteral or mucosal inoculation.

The deceased, and any bagged disposal items, should be tagged as above to prevent unwitting subsequent exposure of other personnel to contaminated articles. Methods that will avoid or minimize aerosol distribution of infectious agents should be used. As an example, bones should be cut with a handsaw rather than an electric saw.

The following should be decontaminated with 0.5 percent sodium hypochlorite at the conclusion of an autopsy:

1. Autopsy table
2. All contaminated instruments, for 1 hour before washing and autoclaving.
3. Other contaminated items that cannot be disposed of or autoclaved, including the outside of tissue containers.

Tissue samples should be thoroughly fixed in 10 percent buffered formalin before trimming for histology.

REFERENCES

Guidelines for the Hospital Care and Treatment of AIDS Patients Greater New York Hospital Association, December 1985

CDC Guidelines for Isolation Precautions in Hospitals Centers for Disease Control, 1983

Summary Recommendations for Preventing Transmission of Infection with Human T-Lymphotropic Virus Type 111/Lymphadenopathy Associated Virus in the Workplace. Morbidity and Mortality Weekly Report, December 15, 1985.

Hospital Care of Acquired Immune Deficiency Syndrome (AIDS) Patients, State of New York Department of Health Memorandum, August 21, 1985.

A Hospitalwide Approach to AIDS: Recommendations of the Advisory Committee on Infections within Hospitals. American Hospital Association, 1984.

CORPORATE POLICIES

The following section contains actual AIDS policies that several companies have developed. They may prove to be a useful resource in developing policies or procedures. These policies have been printed as submitted.

SAMPLE POLICY

LEVI STRAUSS & CO
AIDS INFORMATION SHEET

Policy/Philosophy

> Levi Strauss & Co. does not have a written "policy" about AIDS. The company embraces the following philosophy regarding the welfare of its employees:

> Employees with AIDS or any other life-threatening disease are treated with dignity and respect. The company strives to maintain an open and informed environment for all employees.

> Employees with AIDS or any other life-threatening illness can continue to work as long as they are physically able to do so.

Commitment

> The company has an overall commitment to health education. AIDS is a national health problem and the company feels a responsibility to educate its employees so that prejudice and unwarranted fear about the disease in the workplace can be eliminated

Benefits

> AIDS is treated like any other life-threatening condition in respect to medical coverage, disability leave, and life insurance. As part of its comprehensive medical plan, Levi Strauss & Co. offers home health and hospice care for the terminally ill.

Hiring

> Levi Strauss & Co. does not test prospective employees for AIDS, and there are no AIDS screening questions on employment applications.

Reprinted from *AIDS: Corporate America Responds,* with the permission of Allstate Insurance Company.

Levi Strauss & Co. is an equal opportunity employer and does not discriminate against persons because of sexual preference, age, race, religious beliefs, etc.

Education

The company has undertaken a comprehensive education program to San Francisco-based employees. In 1987, a similar program will be rolled out to field employees. The education package includes a 23-minute video tape, brochures for employees and manager's training materials. Sessions typically include an overview of the company's philosophy about AIDS, a discussion of how the disease is and is not contracted, a review of health benefits available to employees, an update on the latest information about AIDS and a question and answer session.

Guest lecturers including an epidemiologist, local AIDS Foundation personnel and a department head of a local medical center have visited the company's headquarters and have spoken to employees about AIDS as part of the continuing overall health education program. Some of the presentations were either video or audio taped and are available to employees through the company's health library.

Pamphlets, company newsletters with articles on AIDS and fact sheets are available to employees through the Employee Assistance Program (EAP) reference library.

Support Programs

Individual, family, or group counselling is available for employees, co-workers, and families through EAP or can be arranged through outside agencies.

EAP staff has compiled a comprehensive list of agencies that assist people with AIDS and provides this information confidentially to any employee requesting it. EAP staff does department consultations for employees who work with someone with AIDS. Topics discussed in these sessions include: grief, contracting the disease, and visitations.

Employee Participation

San Francisco-based employee volunteer groups or Community Involvement Teams (CITs) have actively been involved with the AIDS issue.

In San Francisco, the CITs designated the SF AIDS Foundation one of the beneficiaries of money raised at a "Fun Run." Also, employees have held flea markets, bake sales, and food drives in order to raise money for local AIDS groups. Employee's gifts to nonprofit, non-United Way agencies are eligible for a matching gift from the LS Foundation. Employees have been making donations to groups/organizations dealing with AIDS issues since 1982.

AIDS Task Force

In 1985, an employee task force was formed to support a broad base of activities around education and other AIDS issues. The group — which meets monthly — is made up of employees from various divisions and departments throughout the company such as personnel, communications, community affairs and operations, and office services.

The objectives of the employee-based task force include: developing a comprehensive Levi Strauss & Co. employee education program; raising AIDS-related issues and proposing suggestions for action; providing assistance to other employers or organizations seeking guidance in developing their own AIDS programs and obtaining support for AIDS organizations.

Financial Support

The company made a $30,000 donation to the SF AIDS Foundation in 1985 for the development of the "AIDS In The Workplace" materials. These materials were presented at a conference hosted by Levi Strauss & Co. in 1986.

The Levi Strauss Foundation and Levi Strauss & Co. have donated or matched gifts totaling more than $85,000 in recent years (including the $30,000 gift previously mentioned).

A partial list of grantees include:
San Francisco AIDS Foundation $51,000
Shanti Project $14,500
Home Care Hospice $10,000
Matching Gifts $12,609

PACIFIC GAS AND ELECTRIC COMPANY POLICY STATEMENT AND GUIDELINES ON AIDS IN THE WORKPLACE

In keeping with two of our corporate objectives to ensure a safe, healthy work environment for our employees and the public we serve, and to prohibit all forms of arbitrary discrimination in employment, we have developed the following policy statement and guidelines on how to handle personnel matters related to employees afflicted with AIDS. The policy statement and guidelines are based on the most current medical information on this subject available. If any significant medical developments occur, we will revise the statement and these guidelines accordingly.

Policy Statement

It is PG and E's position that employees afflicted with AIDS do not present a health risk to other employees in the workplace under normal working conditions. Employees with AIDS are subject to the same working conditions and performance requirements as any other employee. However, if there is supervisory concern that an employee with AIDS is not able to perform assigned duties, a medical clarification examination may be required to determine the employee's fitness for work. Lastly, employees with AIDS, provided that they are otherwise eligible, are entitled to coverage under the company's sick leave, medical leave of absence, disability benefits, and equal employment opportunity policies.

Guidelines

1. Employees afflicted with AIDS should be treated the same as any other company employee. However, if their medical or physical condition affects their ability to perform their assigned duties, they should be treated as any other employees who have a disability that prevents them performing the duties of their job.

2. If a supervisor has a reasonable basis to believe that an employee with AIDS is unable to perform the duties of his or her position, the supervisor must request the employee undergo a medical clarification

Reprinted from *AIDS: Corporate America Responds*, with the permission of Allstate Insurance Company.

examination. The results of the medical clarification examination shall guide future personnel decisions affecting the employee.

3. Employees afflicted with AIDS, to the extent they are eligible, are entitled to coverage under the company's sick leave, medical leave of absence, disability benefits and equal employment opportunity policies. When requested, supervisors and personnel department representatives should furnish information regarding those policies to affected employees.

4. If employees who share the same work environment with an employee with AIDS express concerns over their personal safety and health, supervisors must explain that, based on guidelines issued by the United States Public Health Service and expert medical opinions, casual contact with a co-worker with AIDS poses no threat of transmission. If necessary, supervisors should contact an appropriate EAP counsellor to arrange for more comprehensive education efforts for the work force.

WELLS FARGO BANK

PERSONNEL DIRECTIVE ON AIDS

Introduction

The following outlines Wells Fargo's current policy and procedures for handling employees who have been medically diagnosed or are suspected as having an infection with the AIDS virus, acquired immune deficiency syndrome. Wells Fargo developed this policy in 1983 and continues to medically update it through consultation with recognized medical experts from the San Francisco Department of Public Health, the Department of Occupational Health at San Francisco's Pacific Presbyterian Medical Center and the U.S. Department of Health and Human Services' Centers for Disease Control in Atlanta. Excerpts from this policy will appear in the revised Supervisor's Guide in the Personnel Section.

Purpose

The purpose of the AIDS policy is to reassure employees that AIDS is not spread through casual contact during normal work practices and to reduce unrealistic fears about contracting an AIDS virus-related condition. This policy also protects the legal rights of employees to work who are diagnosed with an AIDS virus-related condition and provides guidelines to manage employees or situations where infection with the AIDS virus is suspected. Wells Fargo's policy encourages supervisors to convey sensitivity and understanding to employees affected with a condition of the AIDS virus.

General Policy

Wells Fargo is committed to maintaining a healthy work environment by protecting the physical and emotional health and well-being of all employees in the workplace. The bank also has a continuing commitment to provide employment for physically handicapped people who are able to work. This AIDS policy is a direct outgrowth of those commitments. It provides guidelines to manage employees or situations when a question of an AIDS virus-related condition arises. There are three major points:

Reprinted from *AIDS: Corporate America Responds*, with the permission of Allstate Insurance Company.

1. Wells Fargo employees who are diagnosed with an AIDS virus-related condition may continue to work if they are deemed medically able to work and can meet acceptable performance standards. The bank will provide reasonable performance standards. The bank will provide reasonable accommodation if necessary to enable these employees to continue working.

2. Wells Fargo provides AIDS education for all employees to help them understand how the AIDS virus is spread and to reduce unrealistic fears of contracting an AIDS virus-related condition.

3. The term "AIDS virus-related conditions" refers to the following four medically diagnosed conditions:

   • presence of the AIDS antibody without symptoms of AIDS

   • presence of an AIDS-related complex (ARC)

   • AIDS

   • central nervous system infection

Medical Overview

Medical experts on AIDS virus-related conditions have informed Wells Fargo that there is no known risk of AIDS transmission between an affected employee and other employees through either casual or close contact that occurs during normal work activities. An AIDS virus-related condition is not transmitted by breathing the same air, using the same lavatories, touching a common piece of paper, or using the same telephone. Transmission of the virus through oral secretions or tears is not a recognized risk according to medical authorities. Additionally, the virus is very fragile and has been found to be transmitted only through intimate exchange of bodily fluids (for example, blood or blood-contaminated tissue fluids such as semen or vaginal fluids).

The AIDS virus attacks the immune system causing a breakdown in a person's normal protection against infection. This leaves the body vulnerable to life-threatening illnesses. In addition, the virus by itself can affect the nervous system.

Individuals of all sexual preferences are at risk of contracting an AIDS virus-related condition. According to medical experts, the AIDS virus is transmitted in the following ways: sexual contact through transmission of semen or vaginal fluids; intravenous drug administration with contaminated needles; administration of contaminated blood or blood products; and passage of the virus from infected mothers to their fetus or newborn. However, there is no evidence to suggest that pregnant women are particularly susceptible to any AIDS virus-related illness or condition. Recent medical evidence suggests that an AIDS virus-related condition can have an incubation period of several weeks, months, or years before symptoms appear. Medical findings indicate that a person who has a positive antibody test will not necessarily develop an AIDS virus-related condition. The presence of the AIDS antibody is a sign of infection, not immunity, unfortunately.

As is true for any person with a life-threatening illness, a person diagnosed with an AIDS virus-related condition deserves and requires compassion and understanding. While that person is attempting to cope with his or her own vulnerability and fears, the support and understanding of friends and colleagues can be particularly valuable.

Some people have fears about contracting AIDS based on misinformation or lack of knowledge about how AIDS is spread. Education providing accurate medical information can best alleviate fears of contracting an AIDS condition. Learning preventive measures to avoid contracting an AIDS condition is everyone's best protection.

Employee Assistance Services will provide, on an individual or group basis, comprehensive AIDS education and confidential medical consultation to all employees.

Supervisor's Responsibilities

The physical and emotional health and well-being of all employees must be protected and reasonable accommodation for the medically impaired employee with an AIDS virus-related condition must be provided as long as the employee is able to meet acceptable performance standards. To ensure these goals are met the following guidelines are to be followed:

1. Any employee diagnosed with an AIDS condition is entitled, as is any other employee, to confidentiality of their medical condition and medical records.

2. When a supervisor, manager, or personnel officer receives information that an employee has or is suspected of having an AIDS condition, the Employee Assistance Services Department should immediately be contacted for consultation.

3. If an employee with an AIDS condition requests job accommodation for his or her medical condition, Employee Assistance Services should

be contacted for consultation and the employee must obtain a written medical opinion that he or she is (a) medically able to work and (b) needs reasonable job accommodation in order to maintain employment.

4. If it is deemed medically necessary, based upon current physical impairment, the manager and personnel officer will work with Employee Relations and Employee Assistance to acquire any reasonable job modification or job transfer of the employee with a diagnosed condition of AIDS.

5. If a healthy employee refuses to work with an employee who is diagnosed with an AIDS condition and is medically approved as able to work, job transfer or other work accommodation for the healthy employee will only occur when medically indicated by written order of his or her physician. The medical order must be a signed medical statement requesting this job change. In the absence of a medical order, normal transfer procedures will be followed. All disputes will be referred to Employee Relations for final disposition.

6. To ensure that employees have the necessary up-to-date medical information to understand how AIDS is spread and to reduce unrealistic fears of contracting an AIDS condition, Wells Fargo Employee Assistance Services Department has developed a program to educate employees about AIDS. The program is available for bank wide distribution by request to Employee Assistance Services: (415) 396-3033 or tieline 396-3033.

A COMMUNITY PERSPECTIVE

The following guidelines were developed by the San Francisco Chamber of Commerce for use in the business community. These guidelines have been printed as submitted.

SAN FRANCISCO CHAMBER OF COMMERCE
AIDS IN THE WORKPLACE
SUGGESTED GUIDELINES FOR THE
BUSINESS COMMUNITY

Epidemics of disease present enormous dilemmas to our society, straining our human, financial, and health resources. Like smallpox, cancer, and polio before it, acquired immune deficiency syndrome (AIDS) and its related conditions are approaching pandemic proportions. The impact of AIDS is and will continue to be devastating. According to the Surgeon General of the United States:

> By the end of 1991, an estimated 270,000 cases of AIDS will have occurred with 179,000 deaths within the decade since the disease was first recognized. In the year 1991, an estimated 145,000 patients with AIDS will need health and supportive services at a total cost between $8 billion and $16 billion. However, AIDS is preventable. It is the responsibility of every citizen to be informed about AIDS and to exercise the appropriate prevention measures.

If we are to overcome the obstacles presented by AIDS and its related conditions, it is imperative that we respond immediately as a unified society. A comprehensive and effective approach toward combatting the epidemic only can be realized through a national effort with the full support, understanding, and informed decision making of the business community.

Any sensible and humane response to the epidemic must be based on accurate information, not irrational fear and discrimination. There is an

Reprinted from *AIDS: Corporate America Responds,* with the permission of Allstate Insurance Company.

alarming tendency to label people as belonging to AIDS "risk groups." This is not only misleading, it is dangerous. AIDS is not confined to any single community. It is not caused by life-style or sexual orientation. It is caused by a virus — a virus that can be transmitted to anyone who engages in high risk activity. Fortunately, by modifying these high risk behaviors, we can stop virus transmission. Unlike many other life-threatening illnesses, AIDS can be prevented.

We are fighting a disease, not people. The business community in America can and must play a major role in creating policies and disseminating accurate information about AIDS and its related conditions.

Any employee with a life-threatening and/or catastrophic illness such as AIDS, cancer, or multiple sclerosis should be treated in conjunction with the principles outlined below. It is our desire that every business in America adopt and/or incorporate these principles into personnel policies and adhere to the content and spirit of the principles.

1. Employees with any life-threatening illness should be offered the right to continue working so long as they are able to continue to perform their job satisfactorily and so long as the best available medical evidence indicates that their continual employment does not present a health or safety threat to themselves or others.

2. Employers and co-workers should treat all medical information obtained from employees with strict confidentiality. In the case of an employee with a life-threatening illness, confidentiality of employee medical records in accordance with existing legal, medical, ethical, and management practices should be maintained.

3. Employees who are affected by any life-threatening illness should be treated with compassion and understanding in their personal crisis. Reasonable efforts should be made to accommodate seriously ill patients by providing flexible work areas, hours, and assignments whenever possible or appropriate.

4. Employees should be asked to be sensitive to the needs of critically ill colleagues, and to recognize that continual employment for an employee with a life-threatening illness is often life sustaining and can be both physically and mentally beneficial.

5. In regard to the life-threatening disease of AIDS and its related conditions, a person carrying the AIDS virus is not a threat to co-workers since AIDS is not spread by common everyday contact. For

this reason, the AIDS antibody and/or AIDS virus status of an employee is not relevant information in regard to the health and safety of his or her co-workers. Therefore, the AIDS antibody test and/or AIDS virus test should not be used as a prerequisite for employment or a condition for continued employment. Knowledge or presumed knowledge of AIDS antibody and/or AIDS virus status should not be used to discriminate against an employee for any reason.

6. Given the irrational fear that AIDS, cancer, and other life-threatening diseases often inspire, the most effective way to avoid unnecessary disruptions in the workplace is to prepare and educate both management and employees before any employee is affected by a life-threatening disease. To this end, employers should implement educational programs based on the best available medical knowledge to understand the disease; what services are locally available to help employees with any medical, psychological, or financial hardships caused by the disease; and what policies the company has in place to cover employees with a life-threatening illness.

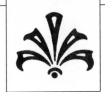

Bibliography

ARTICLES

"AIDS: An Employer's Dilemma," *Personnel*, February 1986, pp. 58-63.

"AIDS: The Challenge to Life and Health Insurers Freedom to Contract," *Drake Law Review*, Fall 1986.

"AIDS: The Corporate Response," *Personnel Journal*, August 1986, pp. 123-127.

"AIDS: Does It Qualify as a 'Handicap' Under the Rehabilitation Act of 1973?" *Notre Dame Law Review*, Summer 1986, pp. 572-595.

"AIDS: The Emerging Ethical Dilemmas," *Hastings Center Report*, August 15, 1985 (4): Supplement 1-31.

"AIDS: Employer Concerns and Options," *Labor Law Journal*, February 1987, pp. 67-83.

"AIDS: The Human Element," *Personnel Journal*, August 1986, pp. 119-123.

"AIDS: It Has Forever Changed the Course of Dental Care," *AGD Impact*, May 1986, p. 1.

"AIDS: The Legal Debate," *Personnel Journal*, August 1986, pp. 114-119.

"AIDS: Legal Implications for Employer," *Michigan Bar Journal*, February 1987, pp. 164-166.

"AIDS: A Mandate for Compassion," *Health Progress*, November 1987, p. 21.

"AIDS: Tackling a Tough Problem Through Policy," *Personnel Administrator*, April 1987, pp. 95-108.

"AIDS and Business: Problems of Cost and Compassion," *Fortune*, September 15, 1986, pp. 122-127.

"AIDS and Employment Law Revisited," *Hofstra Law Review*, Fall 1985, pp. 11-51.

"AIDS and Insurance: The Rationale for AIDS-Related Testing," *Harvard Law Review*, May 1987, pp. 1806-1825.

"AIDS as a Handicap Under the Federal Rehabilitation Act of 1973," *Washington and Lee Law Review*, Fall 1986, pp. 1515-1535.

"AIDS at Work: Fighting the Fear," *Training*, June 1, 1987, p. 60.

"The AIDS Epidemic and Business: A Frightening Disease Poses Delicate Questions for Employers," *Business Week*, March 23, 1987, pp. 122-132.

"The AIDS Insurance Crisis: Underwriting or Overreaching?" *Harvard Law Review*, May 1987, pp. 1782-1805.

"AIDS in the Workplace," *Employee Relations Law Journal*, Spring 1986, pp. 678-690.

"AIDS in the Workplace," *Personnel*, March 1987, pp. 56-64.

"AIDS in the Workplace: Compassion, Not Panic, Is Best Response," *Industry Week*, February 3, 1986, p. 28.

"AIDS in the Workplace: An Epidemic of Fear," *National Safety and Health News*, January 1986, pp. 34-39.

"AIDS in the Workplace: What Can Be Done?" *Personnel*, July 1987, pp. 57-60.

"AIDS Ministry Taking Shape in Diocese," *Health Progress*, May 1987, p. 60.

"AIDS-Related Cases," *Personnel Journal*, December 1985, February 1986, March 1986, May 1986, October 1986, May 1987.

"AIDS — Specter of Fear: Call for Concern," *CMI Journal*, Vol. 10, No. 10, August/September 1987.

"Anatomy of an AIDS Dispute," *Across the Board*, September 1, 1986, pp. 62-63.

Banks, R.A., et. al., "AIDS: A Problem for Intensive Care," *Intensive Care Medicine*, 1985, pp. 169-171.

Brandt, E.N., Jr., "Implications of the Acquired Immunodeficiency Syndrome for Health Policy," *Ann. Internal Medicine*, November 1985, pp. 771-773.

"Comp Board Rejects AIDS Disability Pay," *Business Insurance*, May 25, 1987, p. 11.

"The Constitutional Rights of AIDS Carriers," *Harvard Law Review*, April 1986, pp. 1274-1292.

"Coping with AIDS," *Association Management*, September 1, 1986, p. 39.

"The Cost Impact of AIDS on Employee Benefits Programs," *Compensation & Benefits Management*.

Cowell, Susan, RN, "AIDS and Community Health Issues," *Journal of American College Health*, June 1985, pp. 253-258.

"The Developing Law on AIDS in the Workplace," *Maryland Law Review*, Winter 1987, pp. 284-319.

Dunphy, Richard, "Helping Persons with AIDS Find Meaning and Hope," *Health Progress*, May 1987, p. 58.

"Employee Privacy Rights: Everything You Always Wanted to Know — But Shouldn't," *Michigan Bar Journal*, October 1985, pp. 1104-1111.

"Employment Discrimination Against Persons with AIDS," *Clearinghouse Review*, March 1, 1986, p. 1292.

"Employment Discrimination Against Persons with AIDS," *University of Dayton Law Review*, Spring 1985, pp. 681-703.

"Employment Discrimination Against the Handicapped and Sec. 504 of the Rehabilitation Act," *Harvard Law Review*, February 1984, pp. 997-1015.

"Fear and Loathing in the Workplace: What Managers Can Do About AIDS," *Business Week*, November 25, 1985, p. 126.

"The Fear of AIDS," *Harvard Business Review*, July/August 1986, p. 28.

Graf, Sr. Theresa M., RN. "Unmasking AIDS," *Home Health Nurse*, January/February 1984, pp. 44-47.

"Healthcare Professions Serve as Catalysts in AIDS Education," *Health Progress*, July-August 1987, p. 36.

"How Firms are Dealing with AIDS," *Chicago Tribune*, July 19, 1987, p. 7, sec. 1.

Iglehart, John, and White, Jane, "Policymakers Grapple with AIDS Costs and Controversies," *Health Progress*, December 1987, p. 18.

"Is AIDS a Disability?" *Practical Lawyer*, September 1986, pp. 13-24.

"Legal Aspects of AIDS," *Whittier Law Review*, Spring 1986, p. 651.

"Legal Issues Involved in Private Sector Medical Testing of Job Applicants and Employees," *Indiana Law Review,* Spring 1987, pp. 517-537.

"Levi's Broad AIDS Program," *The New York Times,* March 12, 1987, p. 29.

"Living with AIDS in the Workplace," *Across the Board,* September 1, 1986, pp. 56-61.

"Long Term Care Facilities Opening Doors to AIDS Patients," *Health Progress,* December 1987, p. 22.

"The Meaning of 'Handicapped'." *American Bar Association Journal,* March 1, 1987, pp. 56-61.

Nelson, William, J., RN, "Are We Abandoning the AIDS Patient?" *RN,* July 1984, pp. 18-19.

"Panic Prevention," *Public Relations Journal,* March 1987, p. 18.

"A Practical Guide for Dealing with AIDS at Work," *Personnel Journal,* August 1987, pp. 135-138.

"Privacy in the Workplace: Health and Liability," *Human Rights,* Summer 1987, pp. 45-47.

"Section 504 of the Rehabilitation Act: Analyzing Employment Discrimination Claims," *University of Pennsylvania Law Review,* April 1984, pp. 867-899.

"Twenty Questions About AIDS in the Workplace," *Business Horizons,* July/August 1986, p. 36.

"When AIDS Struck: Two Firms' Responses Might Be Role Models," *Industry Week,* May 12, 1986, pp. 18-19.

"Where 'Boss' Stops and 'Friend' Begins," *Working Woman,* February 1987, p. 70.

"Who Will Pay the Bill for AIDS Treatment?" *Los Angeles Times,* June 4, 1987, pt. 5, p. 1.

AUDIO/VISUAL

"AIDS in the Workplace," AIDS Project Los Angeles, Los Angeles, CA.

"AIDS and the Health Care Worker," Coronet/MTI Film and Video, Deerfield, IL.

"AIDS in the Workplace Program," George Mason University, Fairfax, VA.

"AIDS and Your Job: What You Should Know," National Audiovisual Center, Capital Heights, MD.

"AIDS: The Corporate Responsibility," National Health Education, Inc., Thousand Oaks, CA.

"AIDS in the Workplace: A Three Hour Teleconference," Public Broadcasting System Video, Alexandria, VA.

"Epidemic of Fear — Update Dec. 1987," San Francisco AIDS Foundation, San Francisco, CA.

"An Institutional Response to AIDS," Carle Medical Communications, Urbana, IL.

"The Least You Should Know About AIDS," Accent Presentations, Solana Beach, CA.

"Managing AIDS in the Workplace," Workplace Health Communications Corp., Albany, NY.

"Overcoming Irrational Fear of AIDS," Carle Medical Communications, Urbana, IL.

BIBLIOGRAPHY

AIDS Education: An Annotated Bibliography, New York University, SIECUS, New York.

The AIDS Resource Guide, AIDS Resource Guide, c/o FAPTP, Gainesville, FL.

BOOKS/BOOKLETS

Advice About AIDS: For Public Safety, Health and Emergency Personnel, Seattle-King County Department of Public Health, Seattle, WA

AIDS Project Los Angeles, *AIDS: A Self Care Manual*, IBS Press, Santa Monica, CA, 1987.

"AIDS: Science and Epidemiology," *Law, Medicine and Health Care*, Vol 14, No. 5-6, American Society of Law and Medicine, Boston, MA, December 1986.

AIDS and the Health Care Worker, AID Atlanta, Atlanta, GA.

AIDS Task Group of the American Academy of Hospital Attorneys of the American Hospital Association, *AIDS and the Law: Responding to the Special Concerns of Hospitals, November 1987,* American Hospital Association, Chicago, IL.

AIDS on the College Campus, American College Health Association, Rockville, MD.

AIDS: Recommendations and Guidelines, November 1982 – November 1986, Centers for Disease Control, Atlanta, GA.

AIDS: The Workplace Issues, American Management Association, Publications Division, New York.

AIDS: Employer Rights and Responsibilities, Commerce Clearing House, Chicago, IL.

AIDS: A Manager's Guide, Executive Enterprises Publications Co., Inc., New York.

AIDS – How You Can Prevent Its Spread, Krames Communications, Daly City, CA.

AIDS Legal Guide, Lambda Legal Defense and Education Fund, New York.

AIDS in the Workplace: Legal Questions and Practical Answers, Lexington Books/D.C. Heath, Lexington, MA.

AIDS: Updated Information for Dentist Auxiliaries, Massachusetts Department of Public Health, Boston, MA.

AIDS Services Profiles: The 86-87 National AIDS Directory, National AIDS Network, Washington, DC.

The AIDS Book, Information for Workers, Service Employees International Union, ALF-CIO, CLC, Washington, DC.

AIDS and the Employer: Guidelines on the Management of AIDS in the Workplace, New York Business Group on Health, New York.

AIDS in the Workplace, National Safety Council, Chicago, IL.

AIDS in the Workplace: A Supervisory Guide, National Safety Council, Chicago, IL.

AIDS in the Workplace, Ontario Public Education Panel on AIDS, Toronto, Ontario, Canada.

American Corporate Policy: AIDS and Employment, National Gay Rights Advocates, San Francisco, CA.

Answers about AIDS 1987 American Council of Science and Health, Summit, NJ.

Bader, Diana, OP, and McMillan, Elizabeth, RSM, *AIDS: Ethical Guidelines for Healthcare Providers*, Catholic Health Association, St. Louis, MO, 1987.

Blanchett, Kevin D., *AIDS: A Health Care Management Response*, Aspen Publishers, Inc., Rockville, MD, 1988.

Corlessl, Inge B. and Pittmann-Lindemann, Mary, *AIDS: Principles, Practices and Politics*, Hemisphere Publishing Corp., Washington, DC, 1988.

Coping with AIDS, National Institute of Mental Health Public Inquiries Branch, Rockville, MD.

The Costs of Treating AIDS under Medicaid: 1986-1991, Prepared for The Health Care Financing Administration, U.S. Department of Health and Human Services, Santa Monica, CA.

Facts About AIDS for the Dental Team, American Dental Association, Chicago, IL.

The Facts About AIDS (And How NOT to Get It), American Foundation for AIDS Research, New York.

Infection Control Guidelines for Health Care and Related Workers, Philadelphia AIDS Task Force, Philadelphia, PA.

Kadzielski, Mark A., *AIDS: Legal Implications for Health Care Providers*, Catholic Health Association, St. Louis, MO, 1987.

Legal Answers About AIDS, Gay Men's Health Crisis, Inc., New York.

Legal Aspects of AIDS, Gay Men's Health Crisis, Inc., New York.

Management of HTLV-III/LAV Infection in the Hospital American Hospital Association, Revised January 1986, Chicago, IL.

Medical Answers About AIDS, Gay Men's Health Crisis, Inc. New York.

Teens and AIDS: Playing It Safe, American Council of Life Insurance and Health Association of America, Washington, DC.

Understanding AIDS A Comprehensive Guide, Gong, Victor, ed., Rutgers University Press, New Jersey, 1985.

Understanding and Preventing AIDS, Krames Communications, Daly City, CA.

What Everyone Should Know About AIDS, About Protecting Yourself from AIDS, What Gay and Bisexual Men Should Know About AIDS, Why You Should Be Informed About AIDS, About AIDS and Shooting Drugs, Channing L. Bete Co., Inc., South Deerfield, MA.

The Catholic Health Association of the United States is the national organization of Catholic hospitals and long term care facilities, their sponsoring organizations and systems, and other health and related agencies and services operated as Catholic. It is an ecclesial community participating in the mission of the Catholic Church through its members' ministry of healing. CHA witnesses this ministry by providing leadership both within the Church and within the broader society and through its programs of education, facilitation, and advocacy.

The Conference of Major Religious Superiors of Men's Institutes of the United States, Inc. is an association of the major superiors of religious communities and institutes of men. CMRSMI promotes the welfare, community life, ministry, and presence of over 30,000 priests, brothers, and candidates of 260 religious communities of men in the United States.